CHIARA

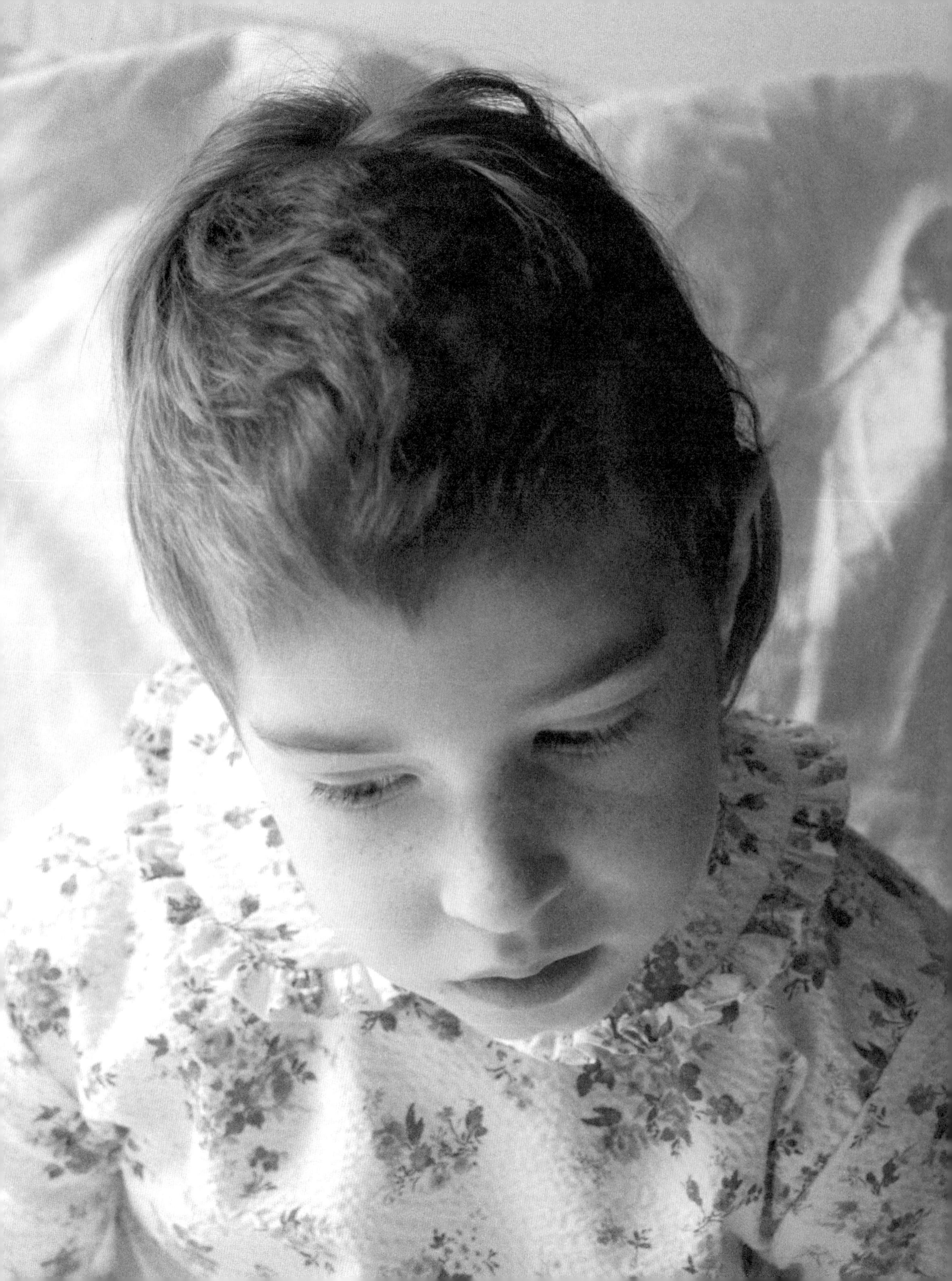

Elisabeth Zahnd Legnazzi

CHIARA

Eine Reise ins Licht · A Journey Into Light

Mit Texten von

With texts by

Nadine Olonetzky

Thomas Macho

Scheidegger & Spiess

Nadine Olonetzky

CHIARA – EINE REISE INS LICHT

Es gibt nur wenig, das schlimmer ist als der Tod des eigenen Kindes. Man hat es geboren oder war dabei, als es zur Welt kam. Hat es gehalten, geschaukelt, gefüttert, geküsst, wachsen sehen. Viele Nächte ist man von seinem Schreien geweckt worden und hat mit einem müden Lächeln über die wachsenden Augenringe gescherzt. Man hat sich geärgert, hat gelitten, ist an seine Grenzen gestossen. Aber insgesamt, unter dem Strich, bleiben Liebe, Freude, Stolz. Dieses Geschöpf, das aus einem hervorgegangen ist und doch etwas ganz Eigenes ist, vor sich zu haben und wahrnehmen zu können, wie es sich bewegt, die Welt entdeckt, zu sprechen beginnt, an Persönlichkeit gewinnt, ist ein Glück, das mit nichts zu vergleichen ist. Man lacht über Ähnlichkeiten, wundert sich über Fremdheiten, man geht mit, wenn das Kind das, was man schon lange zu kennen glaubt, als neu und aufregend erlebt: das Blatt auf dem Asphalt, den Vogel am Himmel, das Feuer im Ofen. Man wird selbst wieder wach für diese Dinge. Von Zeit zu Zeit ist man zutiefst erstaunt, spricht vom Rätsel des Lebens.

Und dann, plötzlich, wird das Kind krank. Keine Grippe, sondern eine Krankheit auf den Tod. Und man muss einsehen, dass die Medizin und auch die Götter nichts tun können, was das Kind am Leben erhielte. Es fällt einem die Aufgabe zu, sein Kind zu begleiten bis an jenes Tor, durch das die Lebenden nicht gehen können, ohne auch zu sterben. Was man an dieser Schwelle als lebender Mensch hart vor

Augen geführt bekommt, ist die Trennung zwischen den Welten der Lebenden und der Toten. Die Toten sind in ihrem Reich, haben dann oft jenen unaussprechlich entspannten, heiteren Ausdruck im Gesicht und sind für die Lebenden nicht mehr erreichbar. Man rüttelt vielleicht an ihnen, ruft sie verzweifelt zurück, aber sie antworten nicht mehr. Der Rest Leben, den die Krankheit noch gelassen hat, weicht nach dem Eintreten des Todes aus dem Körper zurück, verschwindet ganz, und die Hülle dieses Körpers ist irgendwann nicht mehr das Synonym für jenen Menschen, den man gekannt, geliebt hat; sie muss beerdigt werden. Man muss sich trennen. Es gibt keine andere Möglichkeit.

Obwohl wir vielleicht in das gleiche Nicht-Leben eingehen, aus dem wir gekommen sind, schreckt nicht das, was vor der Geburt war, sondern das, was nach dem Tod kommt. Ein Sternchen in der Milchstrasse sei ich vor der Geburt gewesen, erklärten mir meine Eltern, und ich schaute an den Nachthimmel und stellte mir vor, wie ich dort gesaust bin. Warum also nicht wieder Stern werden? Oder endlich Nichts werden? Erlöst sein von den Pflichten, drückenden Lasten, der Bürde des Körperseins (da müht man sich ein Leben lang ab zu überleben und am Schluss ist man doch tot!). Oder in die schützenden, tröstenden Arme eines Gottes sinken, aufgehoben sein in einer grossen allumfassenden, spirituellen Kraft? Dass wir nicht wissen, was kommt, ist beängstigend, eine Kränkung, Zurechtweisung, ein Skandal.

Elisabeth Zahnd Legnazzi hat ihre Tochter Chiara verloren. Im November 1999 – Chiara war fünf Jahre alt – wurde ein Hirntumor diagnostiziert. Der Tumor, ein Astrozytom, war sehr gross, nicht operierbar und er konnte bei Kindern dieses Alters nicht mit Bestrahlungstherapie behandelt werden. Erfolglos versuchte man eine Chemotherapie. Als sich Chiaras Zustand im April 2000 deutlich verschlechterte, gingen Elisabeth Zahnd und Remo Legnazzi mit ihr in die Ita Wegman Klinik in Arlesheim. Gemeinsam mit dem Pflegepersonal begleiteten sie dort ihre Tochter auf dem Weg zu jenem Tor, durch das sie nicht mitgehen konnten. Chiara starb am 17. September 2000.

Elisabeth Zahnd ist nicht nur die Mutter von Chiara, sie ist auch Künstlerin und Fotografin. Das Sterben ihrer Tochter hat sie als Mutter erlebt, erleben müssen. Sie hat aber bald begonnen, den Leidensweg von Chiara auch als Künstlerin zu begleiten. Sie hat Chiara porträtiert, immer wieder. Im Verlauf der Krankheit verliert das Mädchen zunehmend ihre körperlichen Fähigkeiten. Es kann nicht mehr gehen, dann nicht mehr sitzen, irgendwann nicht mehr sprechen, essen, schlucken, es erblindet – nur sein Gehör bleibt bis zuletzt intakt. Doch mit dem Schwächerwerden des Körpers gewinnt Chiaras innere Ausstrahlung an Kraft: Zu sehen ist also immer wieder Chiaras Gesicht, das, oft ungewöhnlich reif, im Lauf der Zeit immer zarter und entrückter wird. Zu sehen ist auch ihr Körper, zuerst noch sitzend, dann mehr und mehr liegend, immer dünner, durchsichtiger werdend. Am Schluss liegt die tote Chiara da, ruhig, weiss, in der anderen Welt angekommen.

Eingebettet in die Umgebung des Zimmers und der Kissen, zuweilen mit dem Vater oder mit der Mutter und Künstlerin im Bild, steht Chiara im Zentrum dieser Fotoserie. Nie haben Elisabeth Zahnds Bilder etwas Reisserisches, nie hat sie diesen Tod in irgendeiner Weise für ihr künstlerisches Projekt benutzt. Sensibel geht sie mit Chiara mit, beobachtet sie liebevoll, und obwohl sie auch nah herangeht, bleibt Respekt, ja Diskretion bestehen. Unscharf aufgenommene, ins Abstrakte gehende Landschaften bringen das Schwinden ihrer Sinneswahrnehmungen zum Ausdruck, öffnen den Blick auf Ungewisses, Entferntes.

Elisabeth Zahnd wandert auf einer sehr feinen Linie, die zwischen allzu grosser Nähe und allzu kühler Distanznahme gezogen ist. Indem sie Chiara zeigt, wie sie durch die Krankheit schwächer wird und gleichzeitig einen Blick zu gewinnen scheint für diese den Lebenden verwehrte Welt, versucht sie diesen Abschied zu erfassen, festzuhalten und damit ein Stück weit zu verarbeiten. Es ist ein stilles Drama, das sich vor den Augen der Betrachtenden abspielt und das zugleich den Mut offenbart, über dieses so oft verdrängte Thema in Bildern zu sprechen. Elisabeth Zahnd vermittelt so, was sie selbst auf diesem Weg erfahren hat: dass die Krankheit auf den Tod auch Lebenszeit ist. Eine Lebenszeit, an deren Ende der Tod steht, und die trotz Schmerz, Leiden und absehbarer Trennung (oder gerade deswegen) intensiv und lebendig ist, voller Zärtlichkeit, Nähe, Wärme. Das, was diese Bilder zeigen, ist eine sehr harte Wirklichkeit, aber sie ist nicht nur schrecklich. Sie ist auch hell. In ihr gibt es das Licht, in das Chiara irgendwann ganz einging. Der Tod ist auch das Leben.

Nadine Olonetzky

CHIARA – A JOURNEY INTO LIGHT

There are very few things worse than the death of one's own child. Either you have given birth or were there at the birth. You have held, rocked, fed, kissed, and watched your child grow. You've been woken up night after night by crying and have smiled tiredly, joking about the deepening rings under your eyes. You've gotten angry, suffered, confronted your borders. But as a whole, in the end sum remain love, pleasure, and pride. It is an incomparable joy to behold this creation, which although emerging from you, is nonetheless entirely his or her own being; to perceive her, how she moves, discovers the world, begins to speak, and develops a personality. You laugh about the similarities, marvel at the strangeness. You are swept along when your child experiences as new and exciting things that you've known about for ages: a leaf on the street, a bird in the sky, a fire in the oven. You awaken to these things again. From time to time you are deeply amazed; you speak of the mystery of life.

And then, suddenly, the child becomes ill. It is a terminal illness, not the flu. You have to accept that neither medical science nor any god can do anything to keep the child alive. You are assigned the task of accompanying your child to that door through which living beings are barred before death. At this threshold, living people are confronted with the harsh reality of the separation of the worlds of the living and the dead. The dead are in their realm, often with that inexpressibly relaxed, blithe expression on their faces, beyond the grasp of the living. You shake them, perhaps frantically call their names, but there is no longer any reply. Upon the entry of death, all remnants of life that the illness has left behind recede from the body; disappear completely. The shell of this body is at some point no longer synonymous with that person that one knew and loved; it must be buried. You have to part from them. There is no other possibility.

Although perhaps we enter into the same non-life from whence we came, it is whatever comes after death that frightens us, not what was before birth. My parents explained to me that before birth I was a star in the milky way, and I looked into the nighttime sky and imagined how I sped here. Why not become a star again? Or, finally be nothing? Released from the duties, pressures, and burdens of physical existence (one struggles a life long to survive and in the end, still, one is dead!). Or in the protective, consoling arms of a god, saved in a great, all-encompassing spiritual power? The fact that we do not know what awaits us is alarming, a slight, a rebuke, a scandal.

Elisabeth Zahnd Legnazzi lost her daughter Chiara. In November 1999 when Chiara was five years old she was diagnosed with a brain tumor. The tumor, an astrocytoma, was extremely large and inoperable and could not be treated with radiation in a child of this age. They tried chemotherapy with no success. As Chiara's condition was clearly deteriorating, in April 2000, Elisabeth Zahnd and Remo Legnazzi went with her to the Ita Wegman Clinic in Arlesheim. Together with the nursing staff, they went with their daughter along the path to that door through which they could no longer accompany her. Chiara died on 17 September 2000.

Elisabeth Zahnd, Chiara's mother, is also an artist and photographer. As a mother, she experienced, had to experience, the death of her daughter. However, she soon began to follow Chiara's ordeal also in her role as an artist. She portrayed Chiara again and again. Over the course of her illness, the child increasingly lost her physical abilities. She could no longer walk, then no longer sit, and at some point she could no longer talk, eat, swallow, or see—only her hearing remained intact until the end. However, as her body weakened, Chiara's inner radiance became ever more intense: visible over and over is Chiara's face, often unusually mature, as it becomes increasingly fragile and withdrawn over the course of time. Her body is also visible, first sitting, then more often lying, growing thinner and more transparent. In the end, Chiara lies there, dead, calm, white, having arrived in the other world.

Chiara is the focus of this photo series, embedded in the surroundings of the room and the pillow, at times with the father or the mother and artist in the picture. Elisabeth Zahnd's pictures have nothing sensational about them; she never used this death in any way for her artistic project. She accompanies Chiara sensitively, lovingly, and although she approaches her quite closely, respect and even discretion remain intact. Out of focus landscapes that become ever more abstract express the loss of the child's senses, open up a view of the unknown, remote.

Elisabeth Zahnd treads a very fine line that stretches between getting too close and keeping too cool of a distance. By showing how Chiara becomes weaker through the illness and at the same time seems to have gained a perspective on this world that is inaccessible for the living, she attempts to grasp the departure, record it, and thereby work through it somewhat. It is a silent drama playing out before the eyes of the beholders, displaying the courage to speak in pictures about this so often suppressed theme. In this way, Elisabeth Zahnd mediates what she experienced personally along this path: that a terminal illness is also life time. A time of life whose end is in death, and which despite pain, suffering, and imminent separation (or perhaps precisely for that reason), is intensive and vital, full of tenderness, closeness, and warmth. What these pictures show is a very harsh reality, but it is more than simply morbid. It is also lucid. In it is the light that Chiara at some point enters completely. Death is also life.

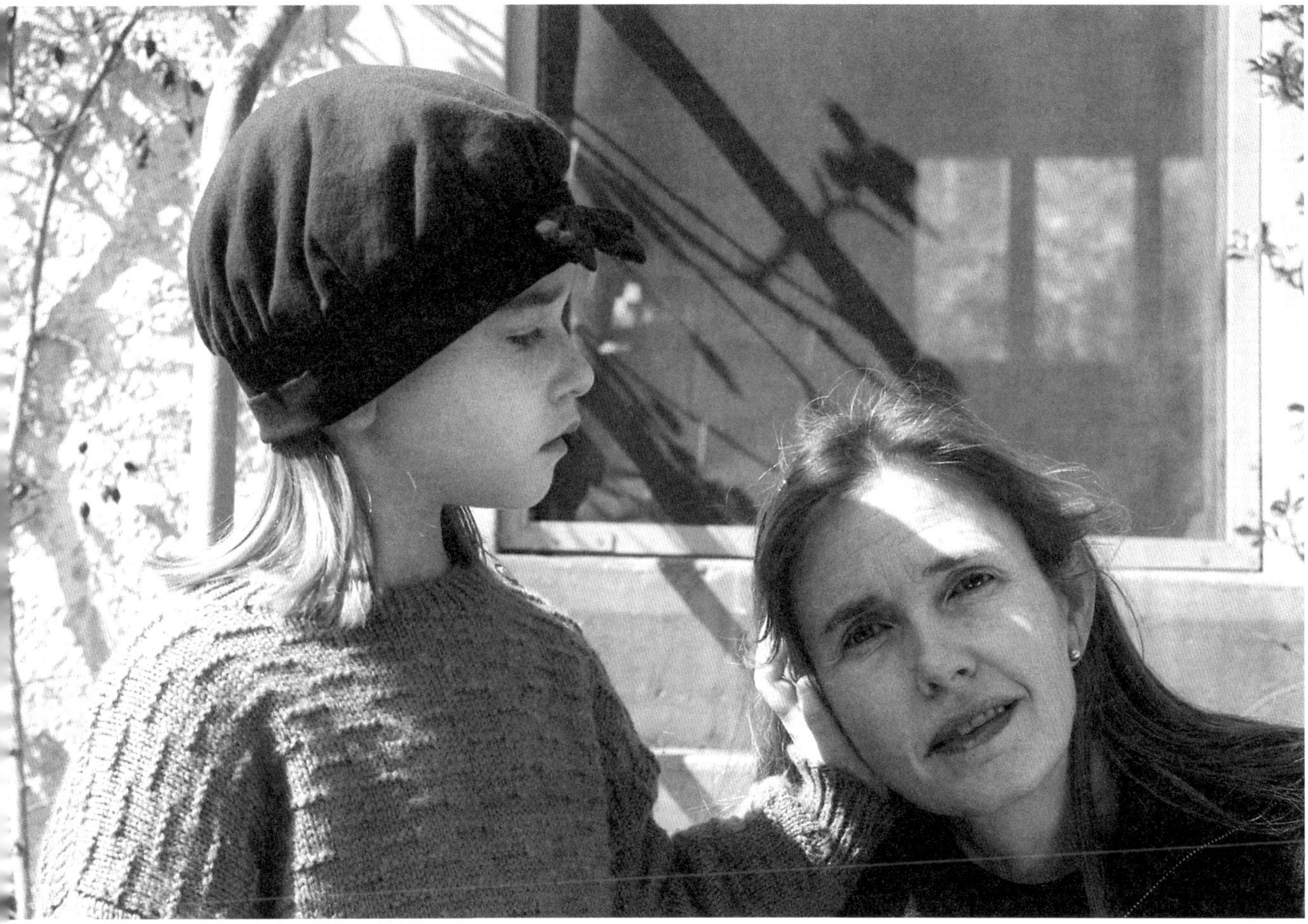

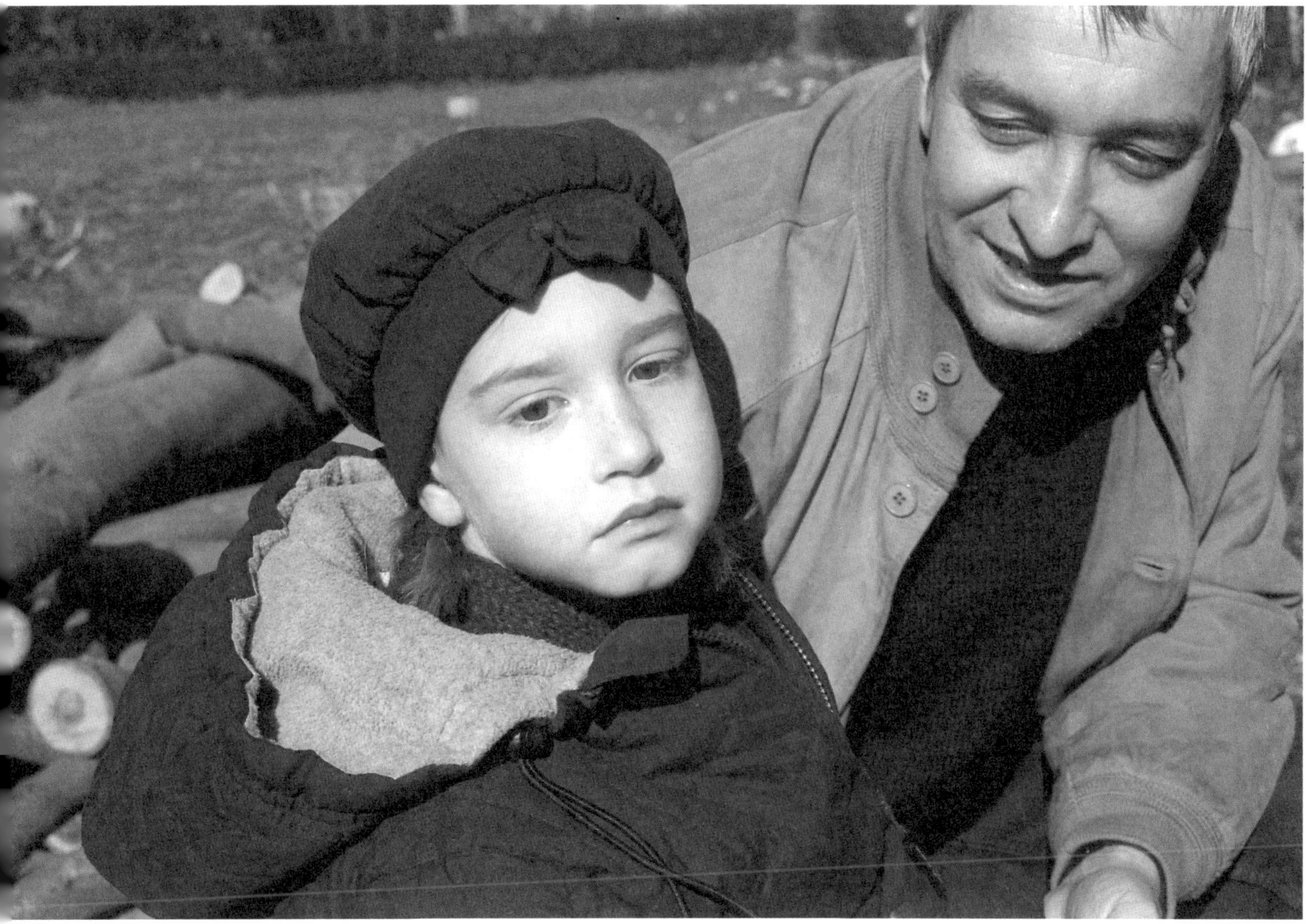

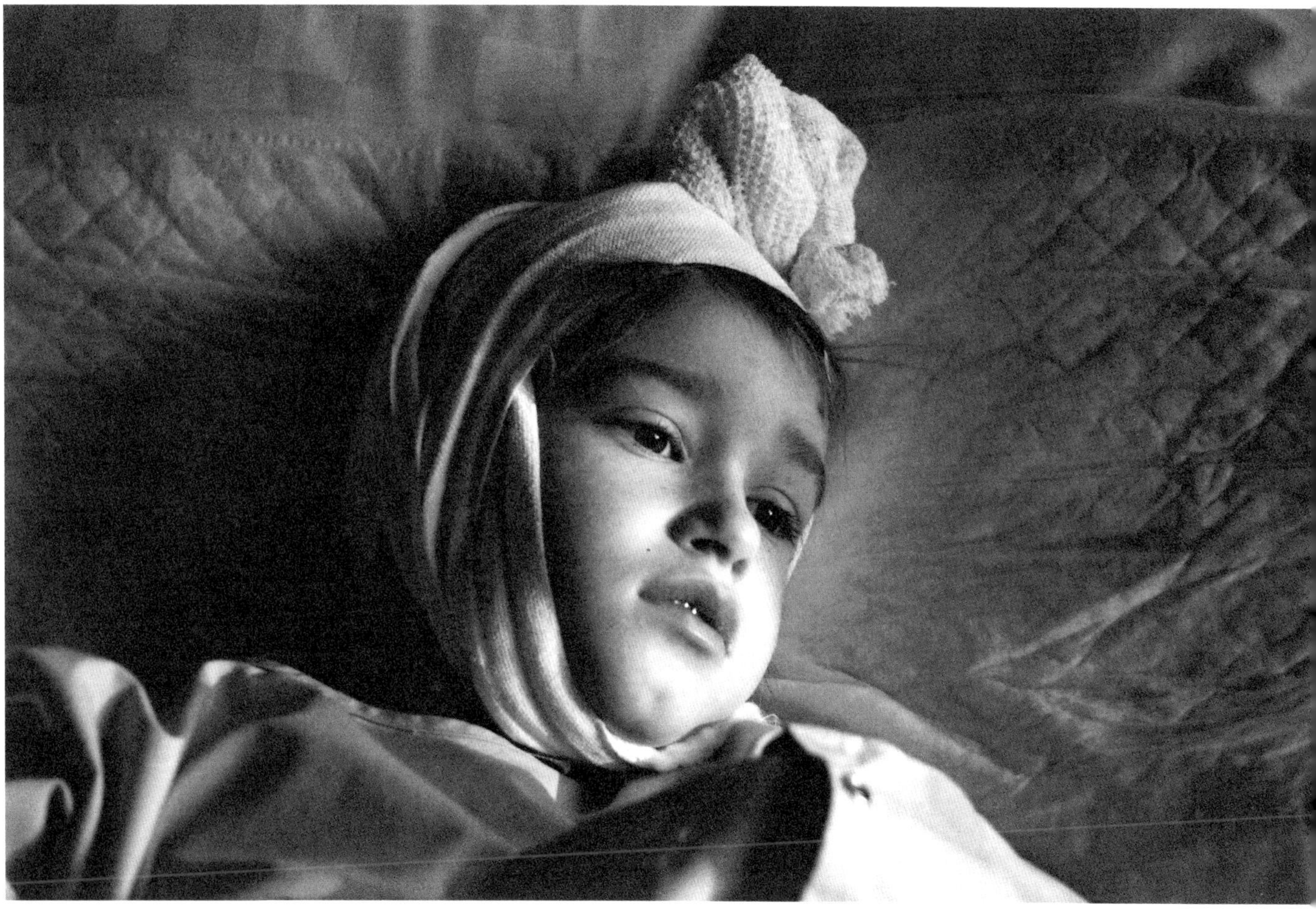

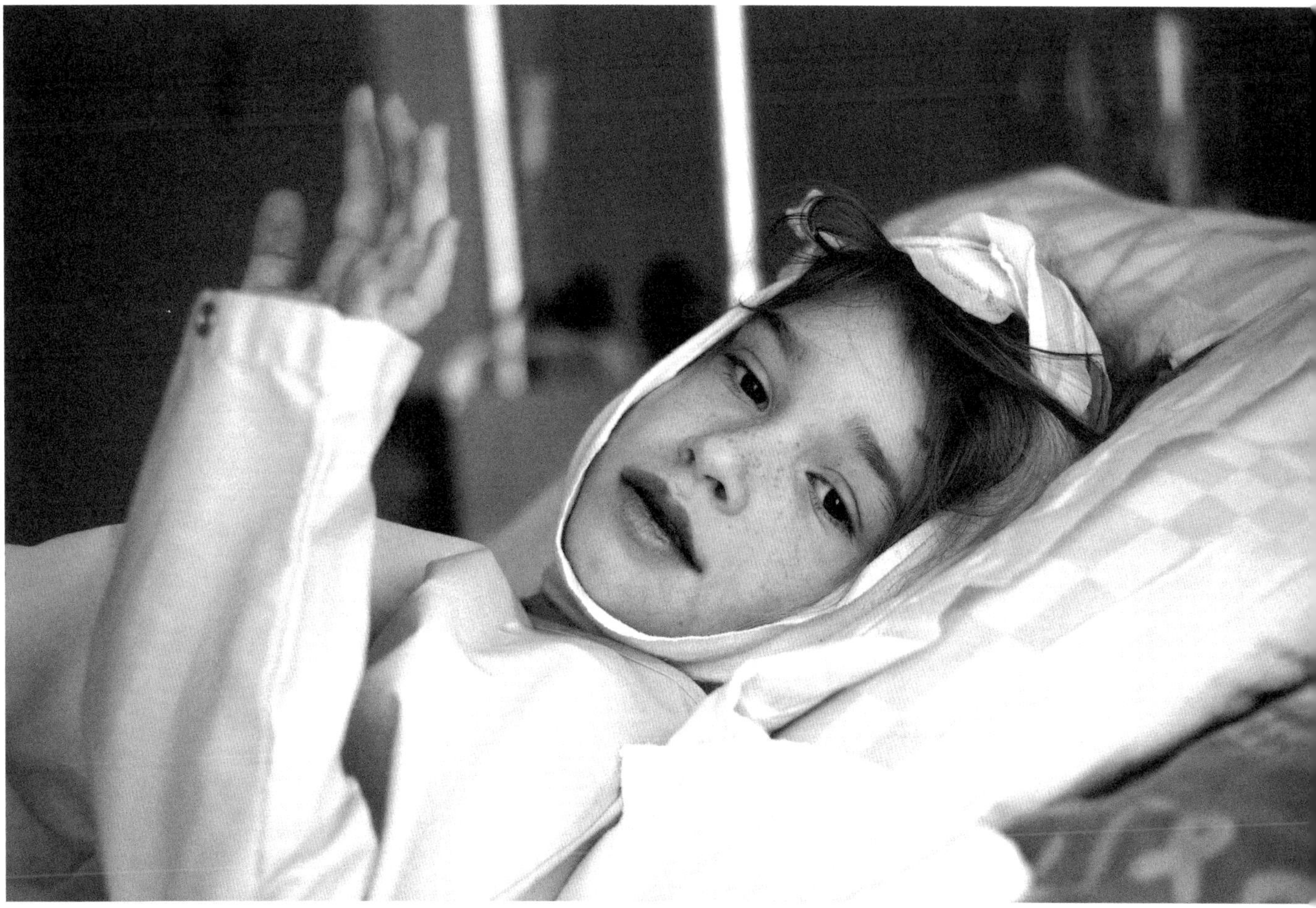

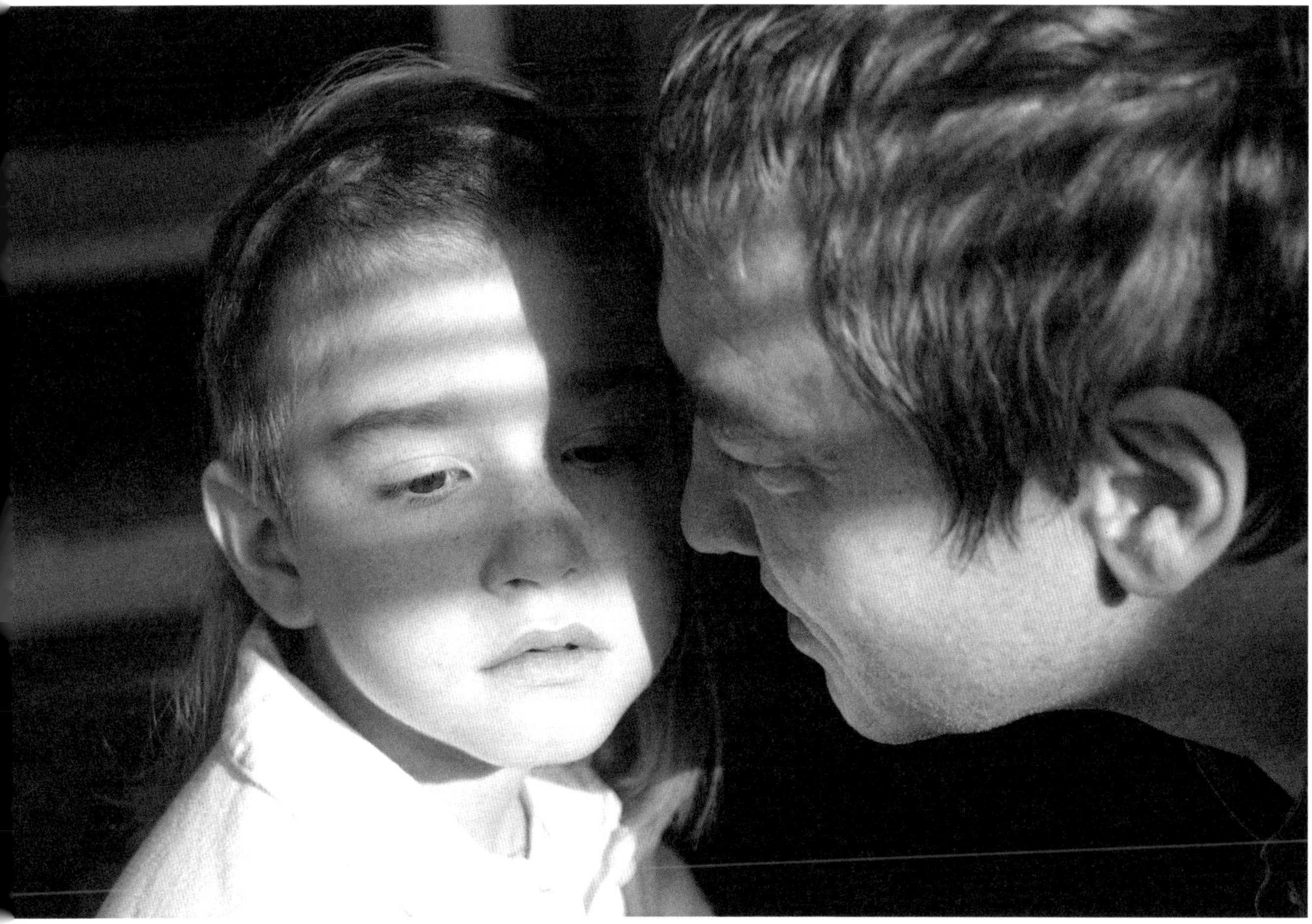

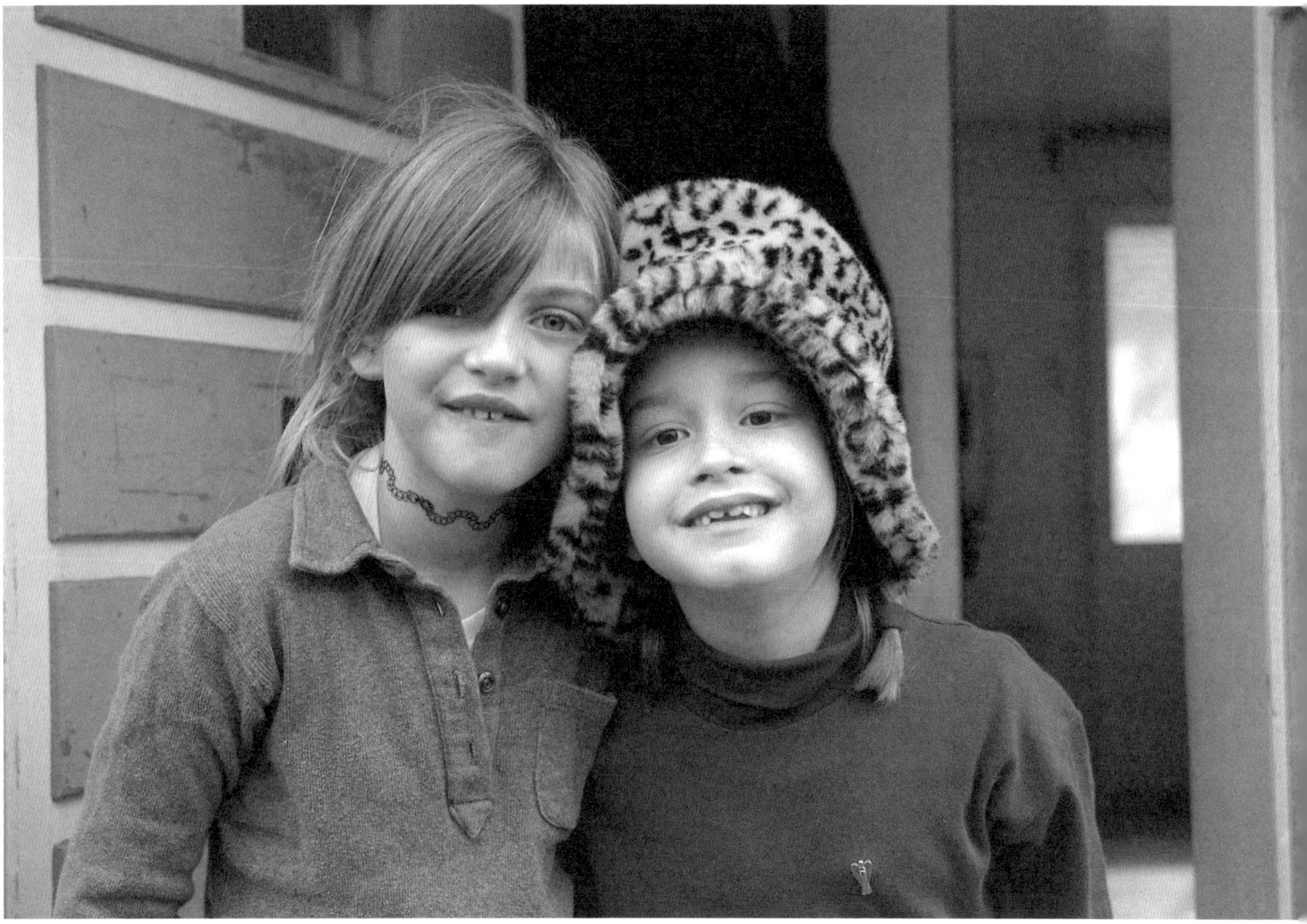

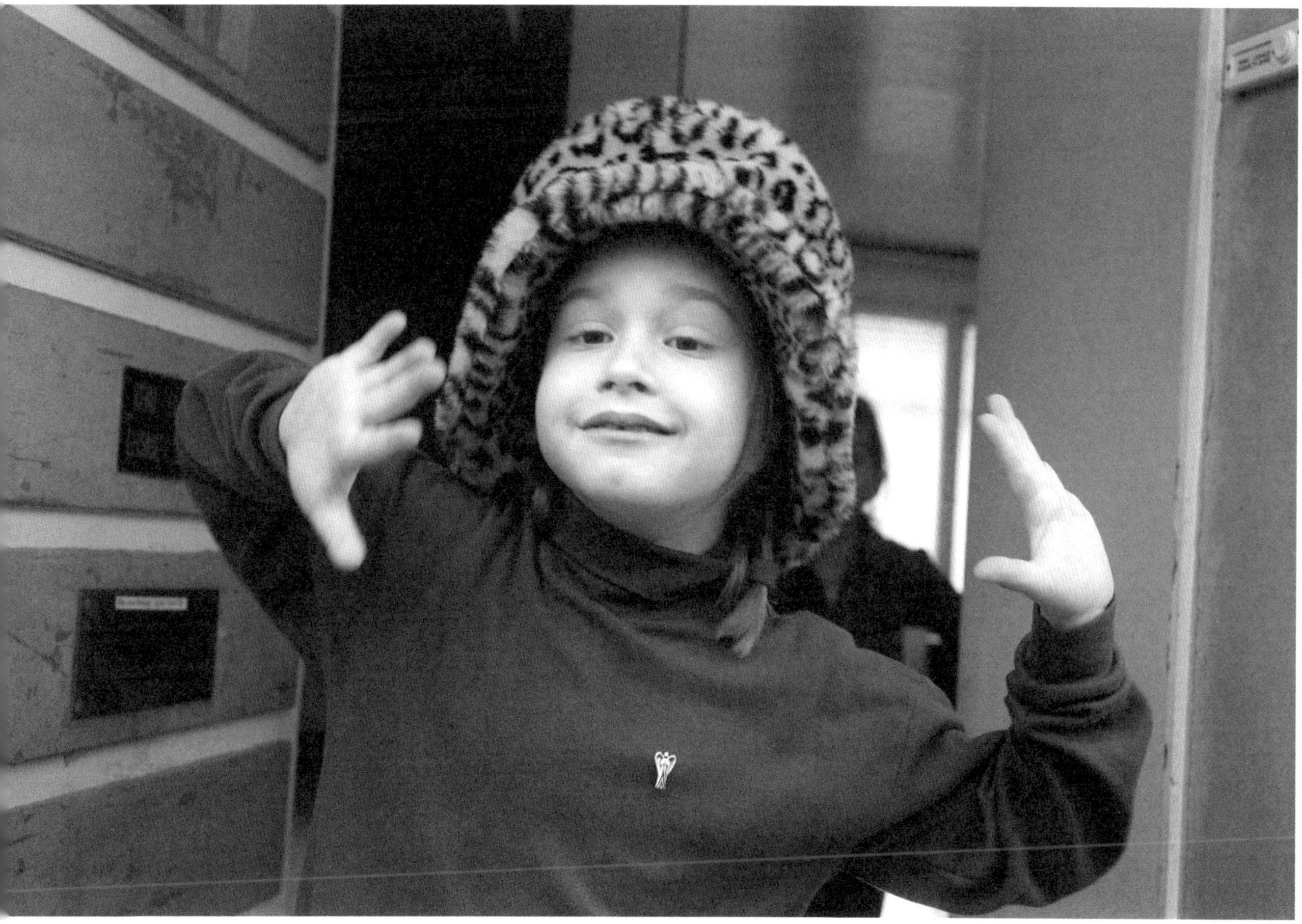

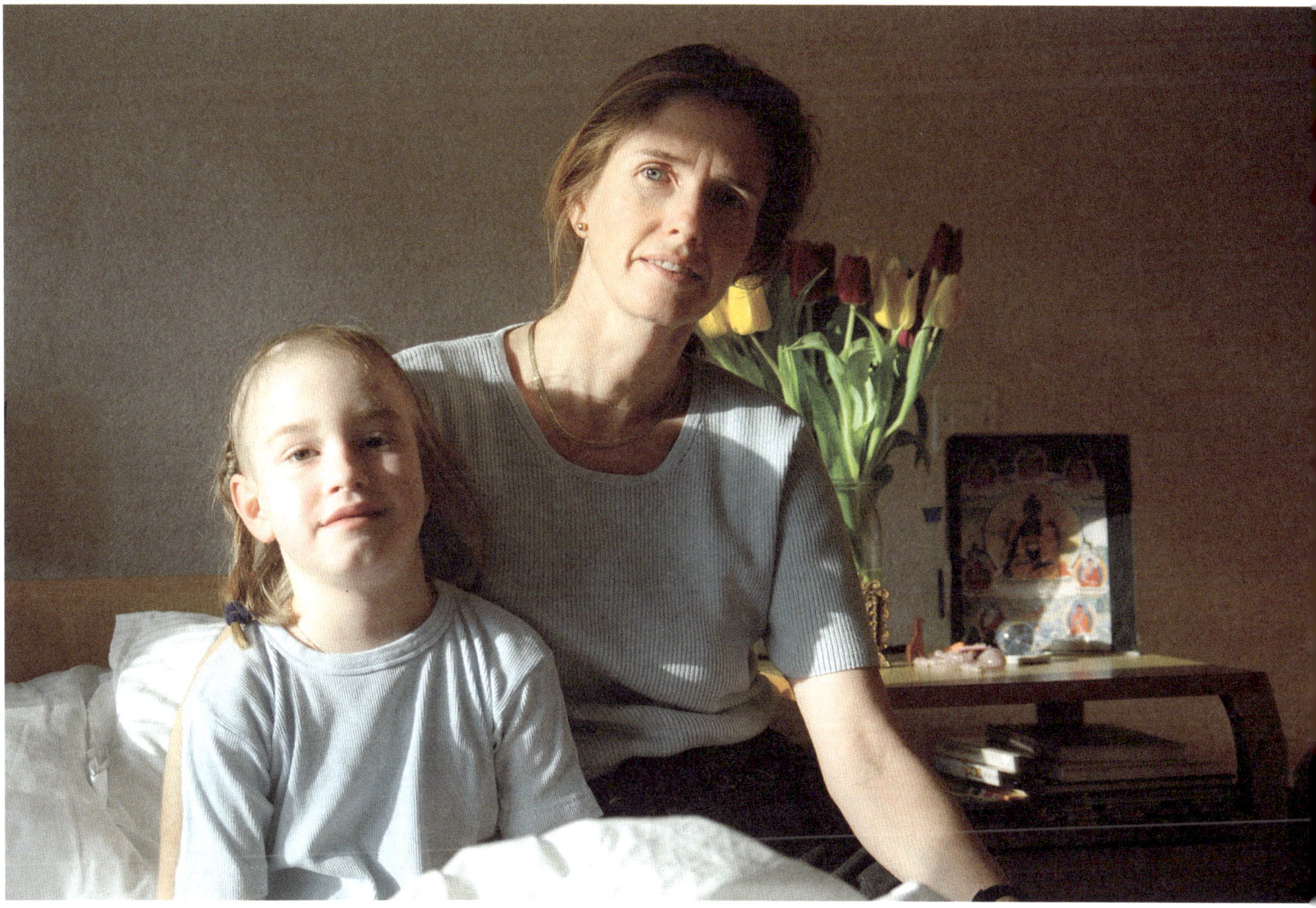

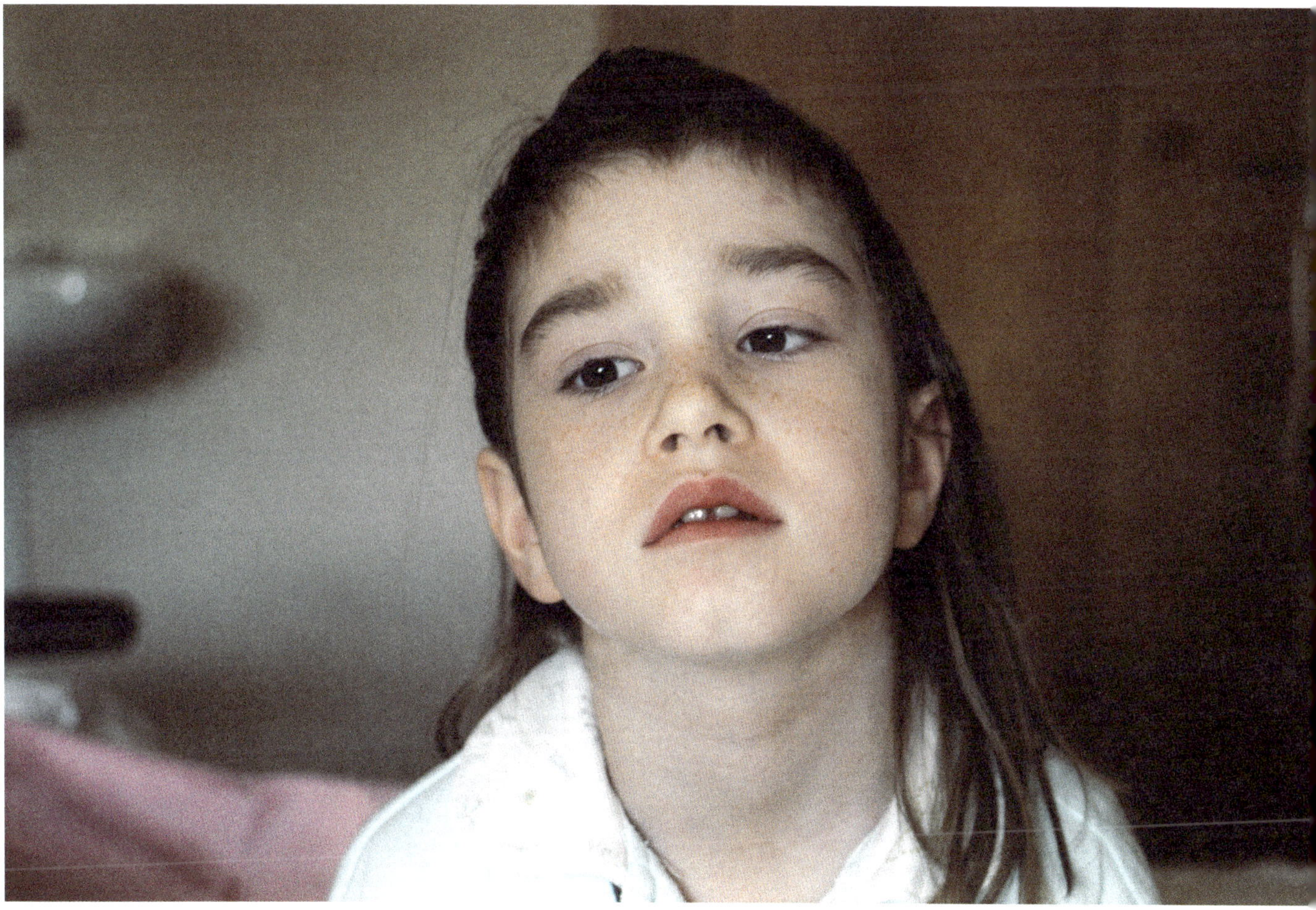

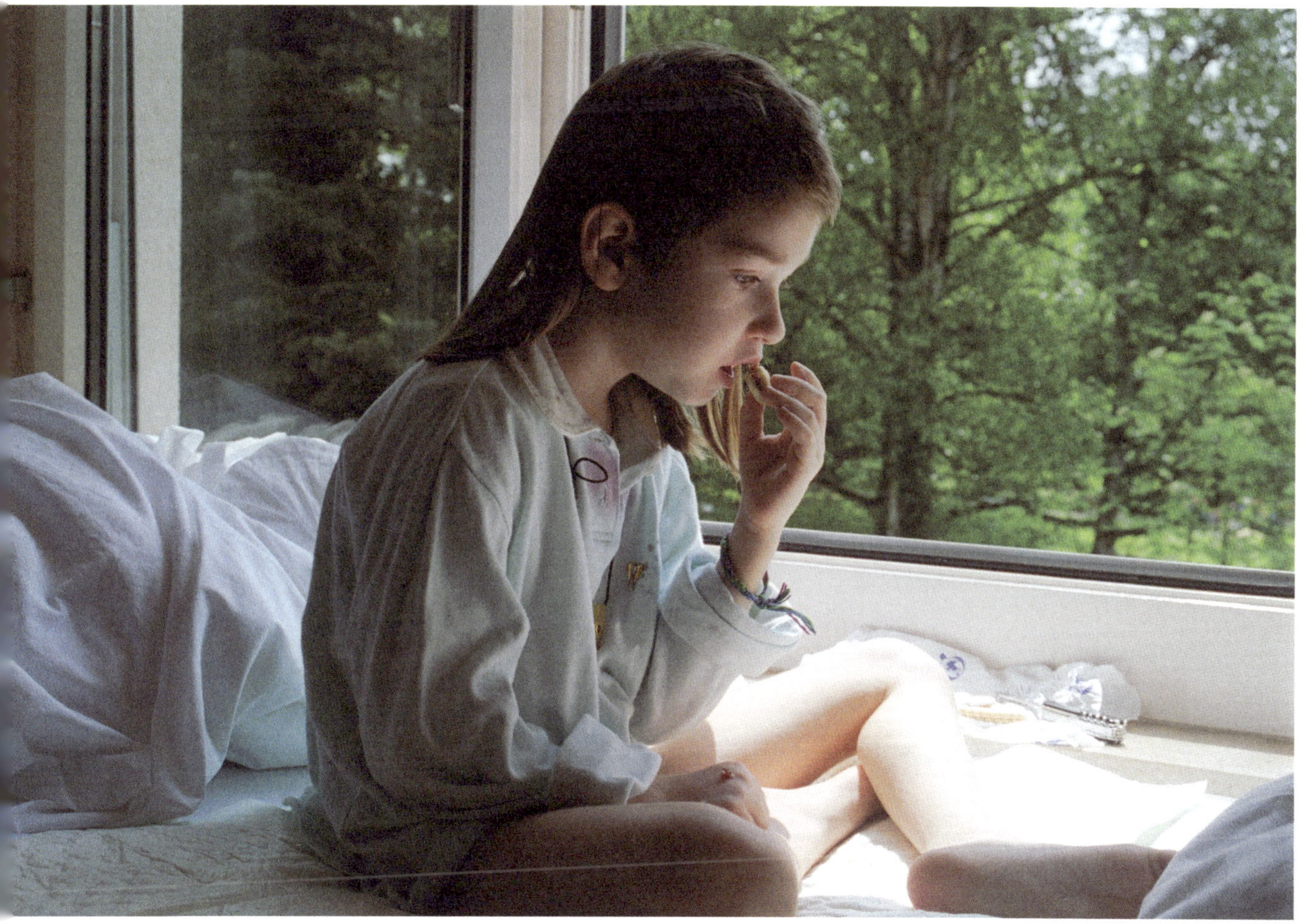

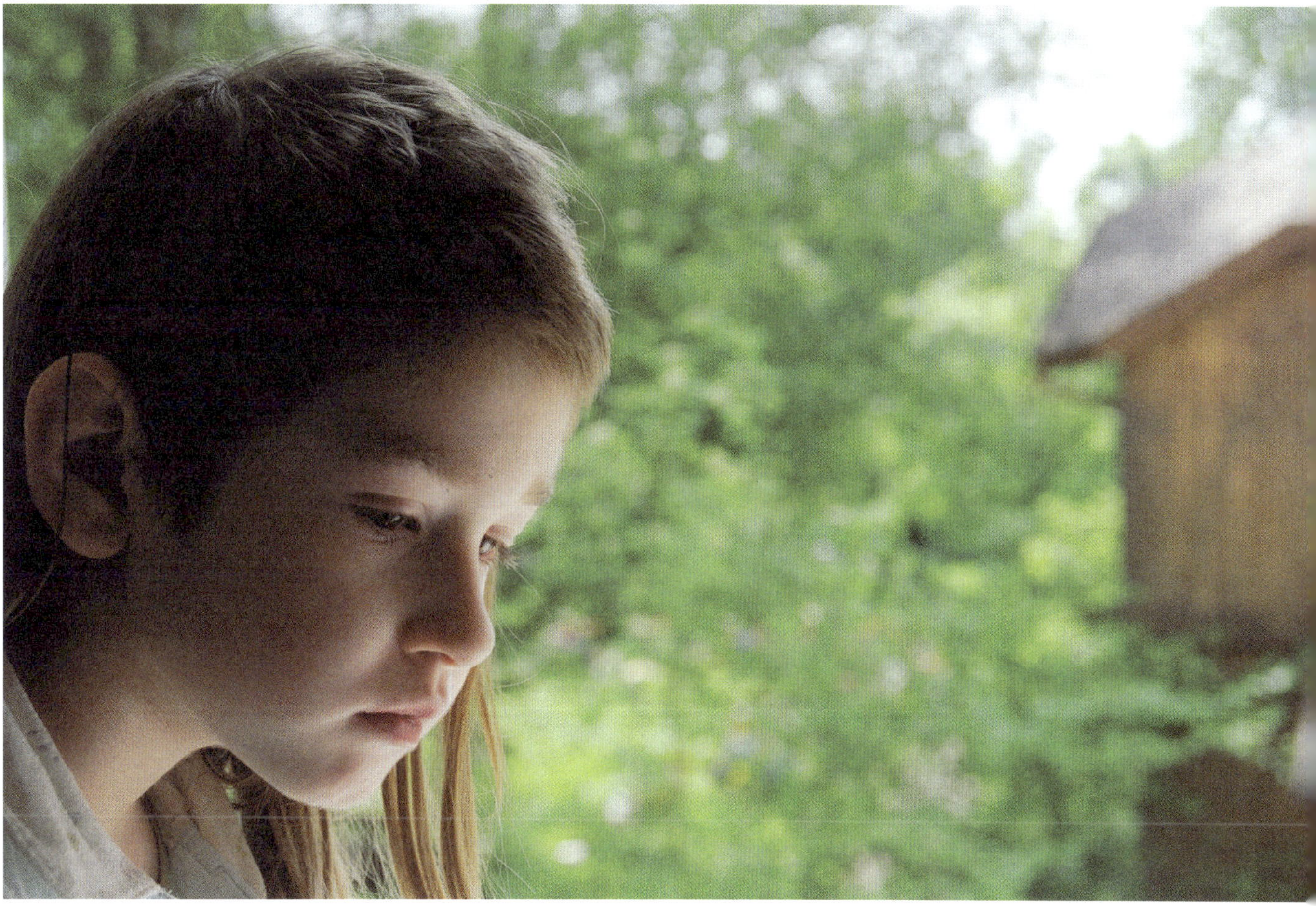

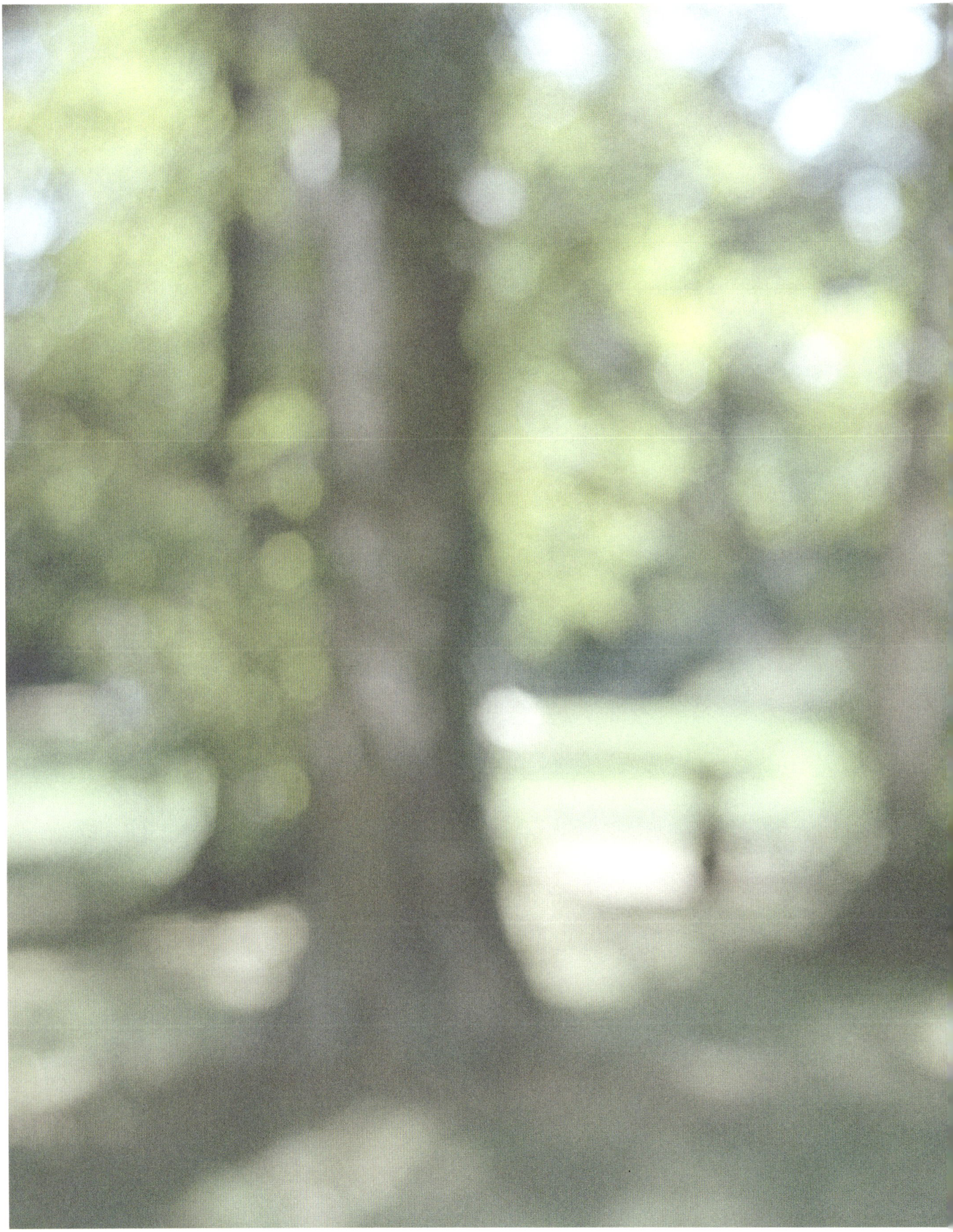

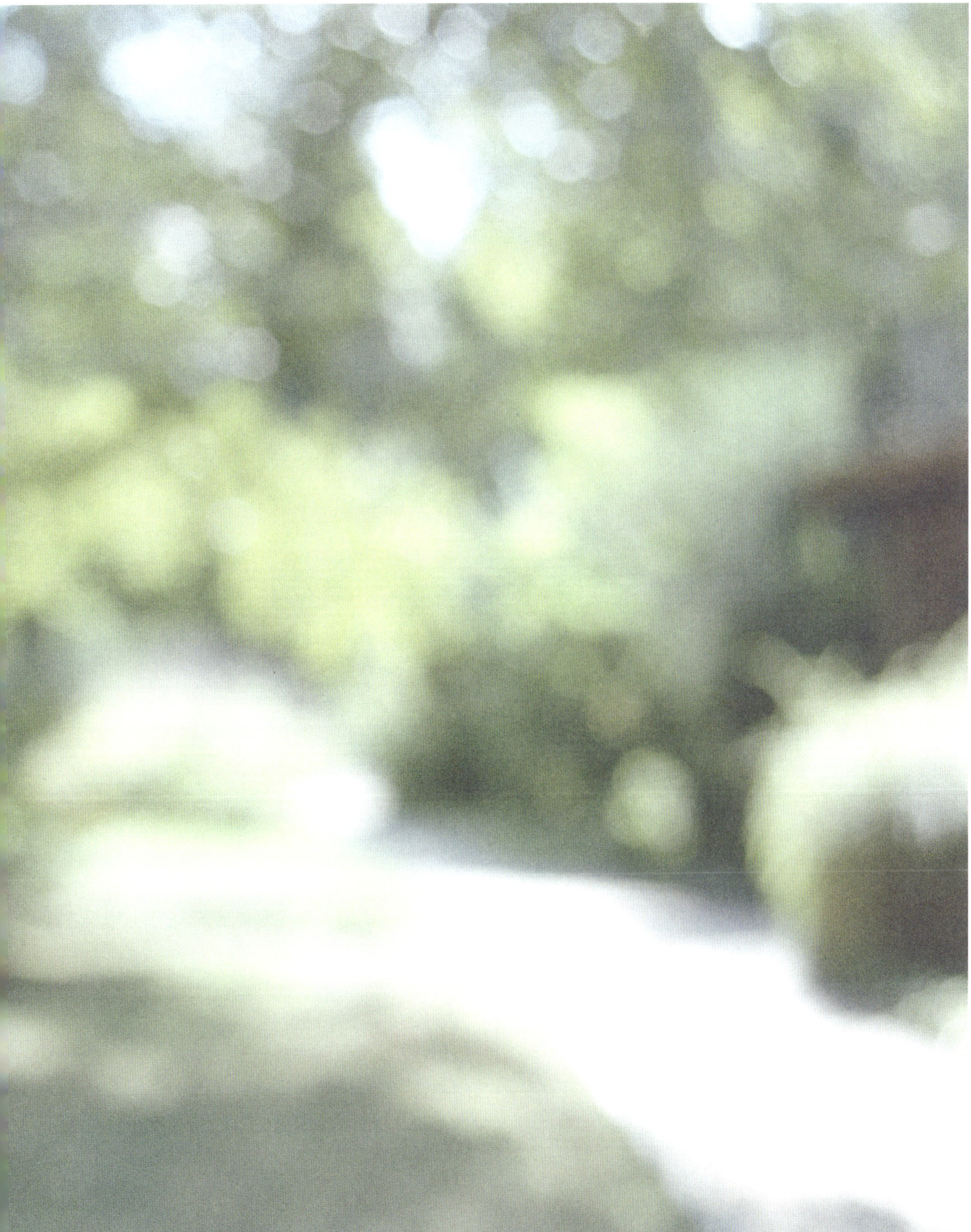

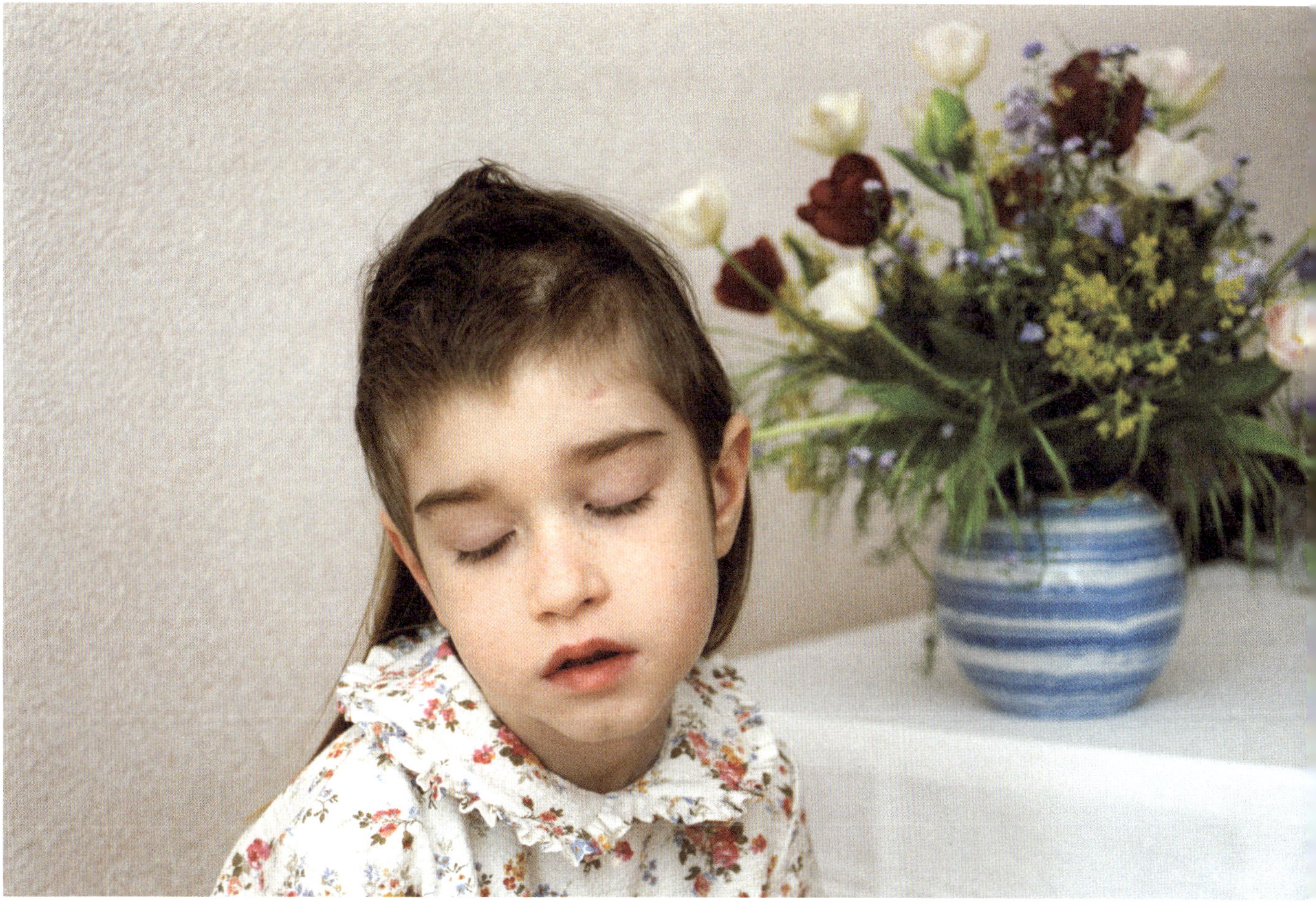

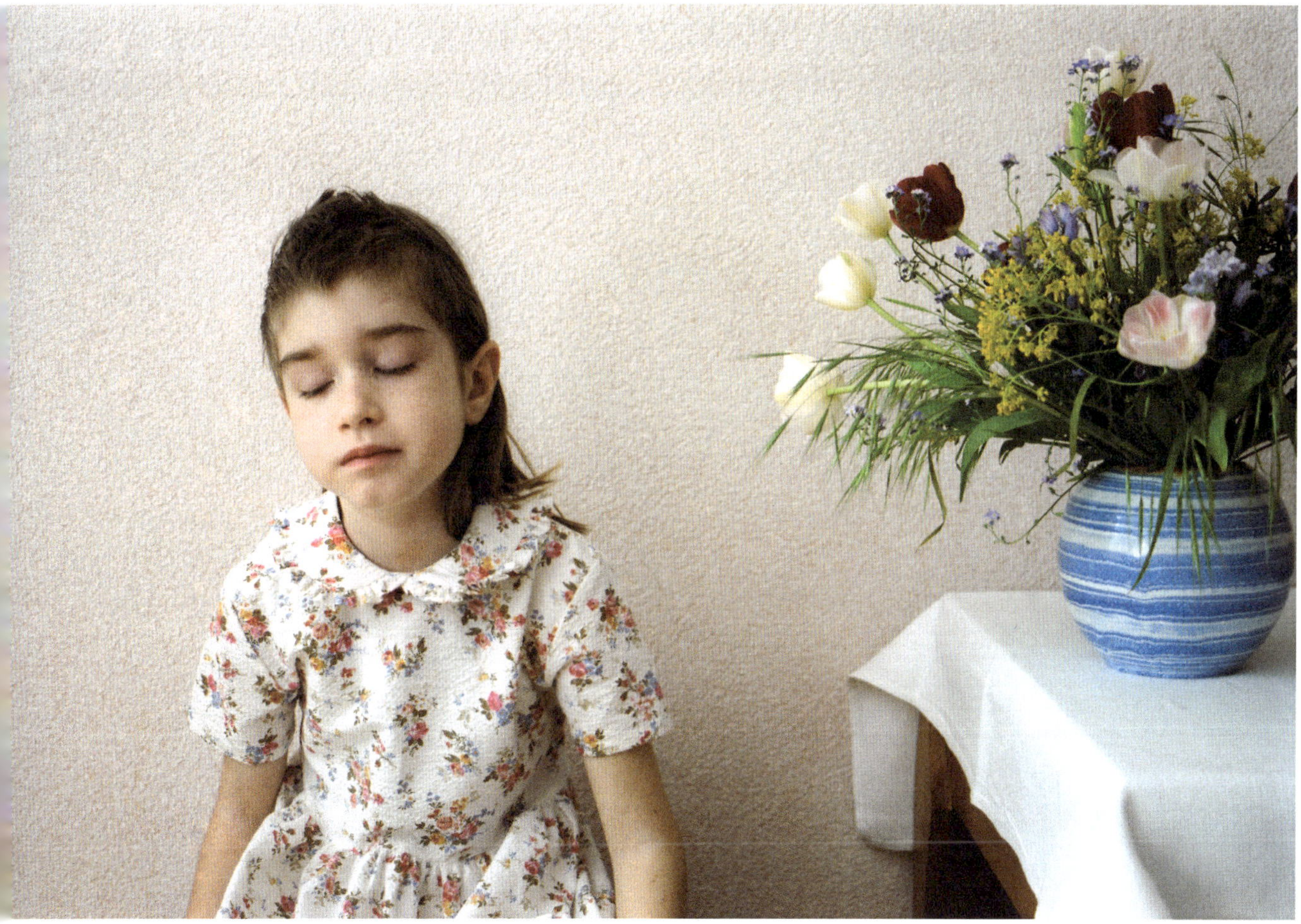

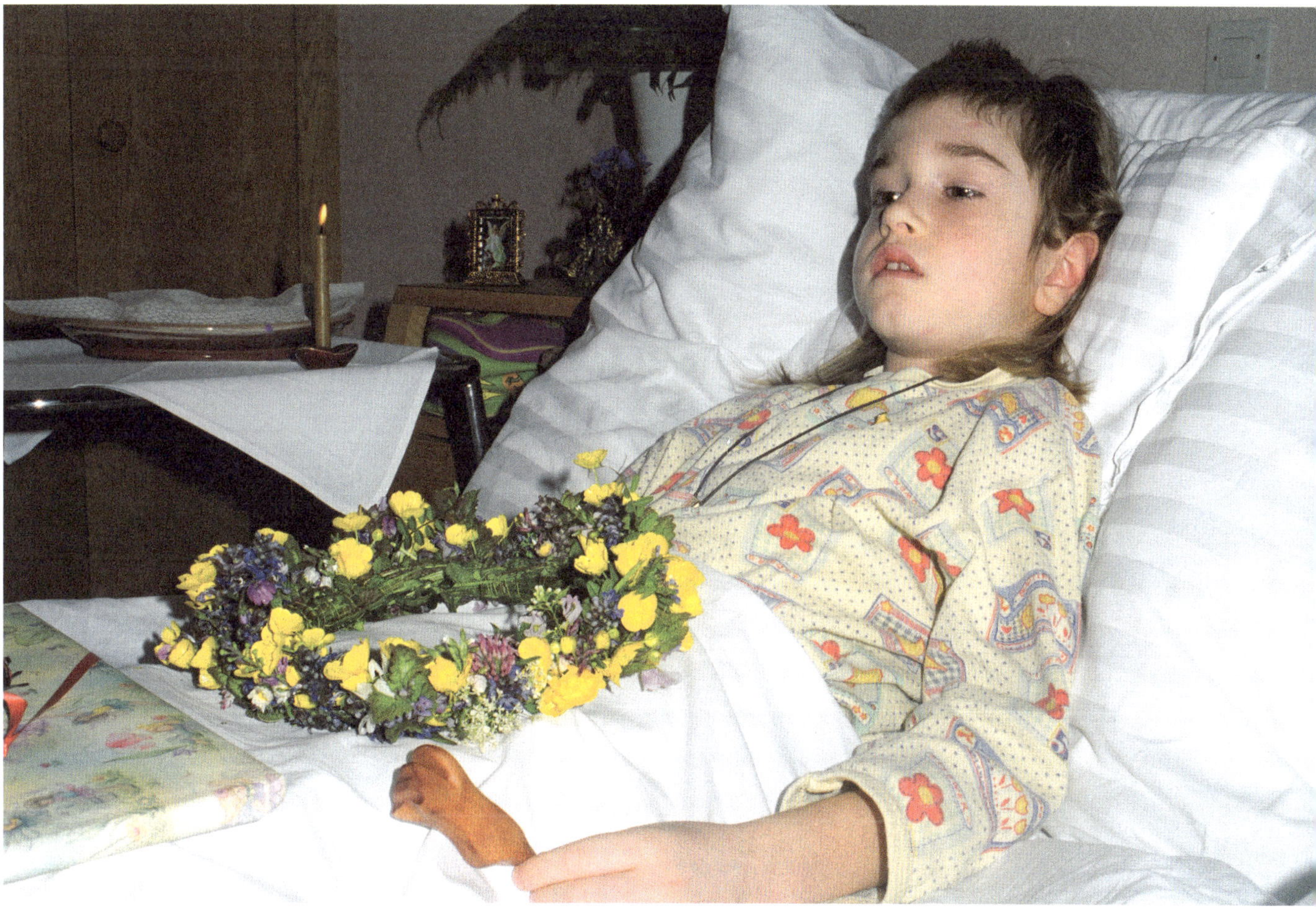

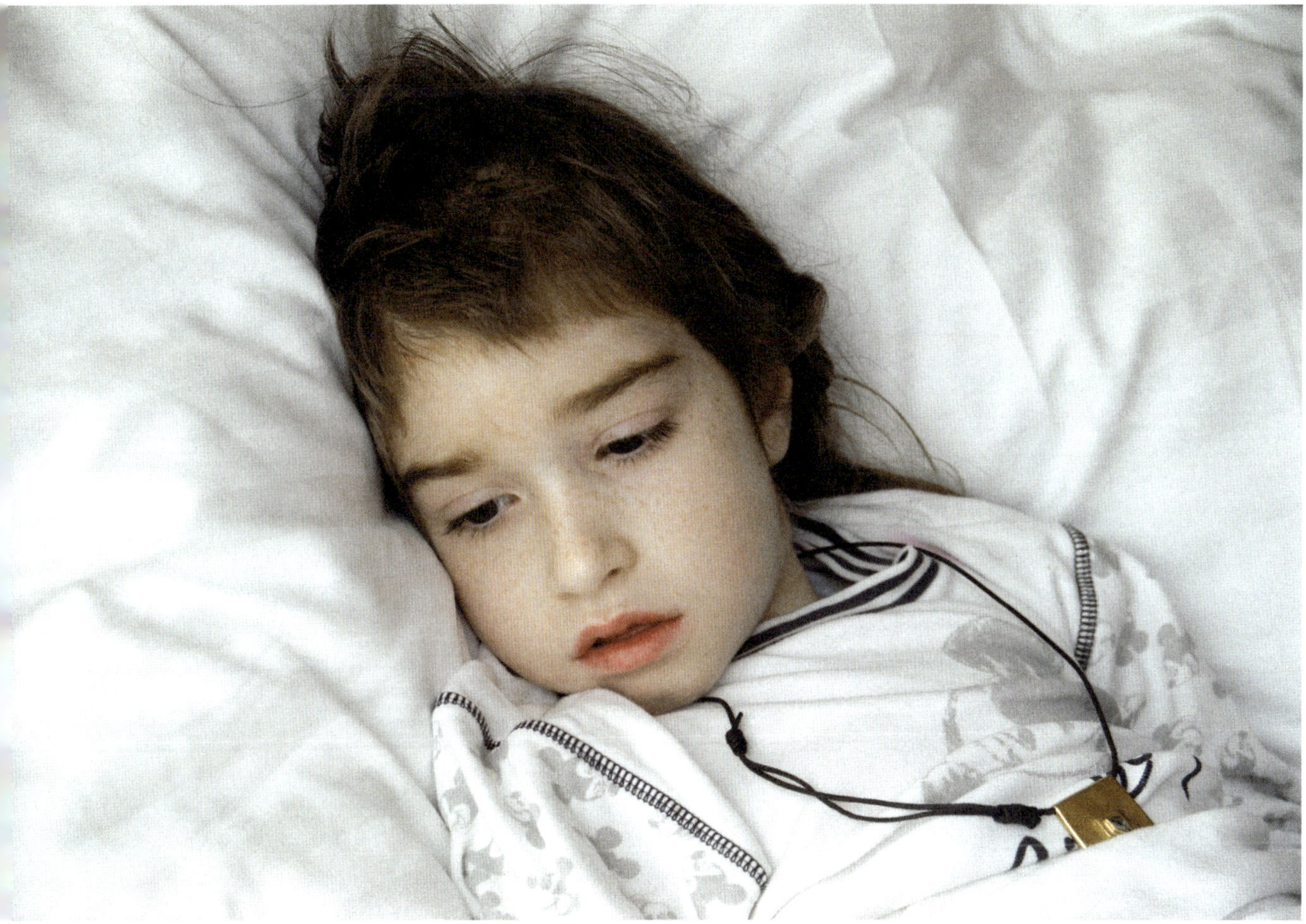

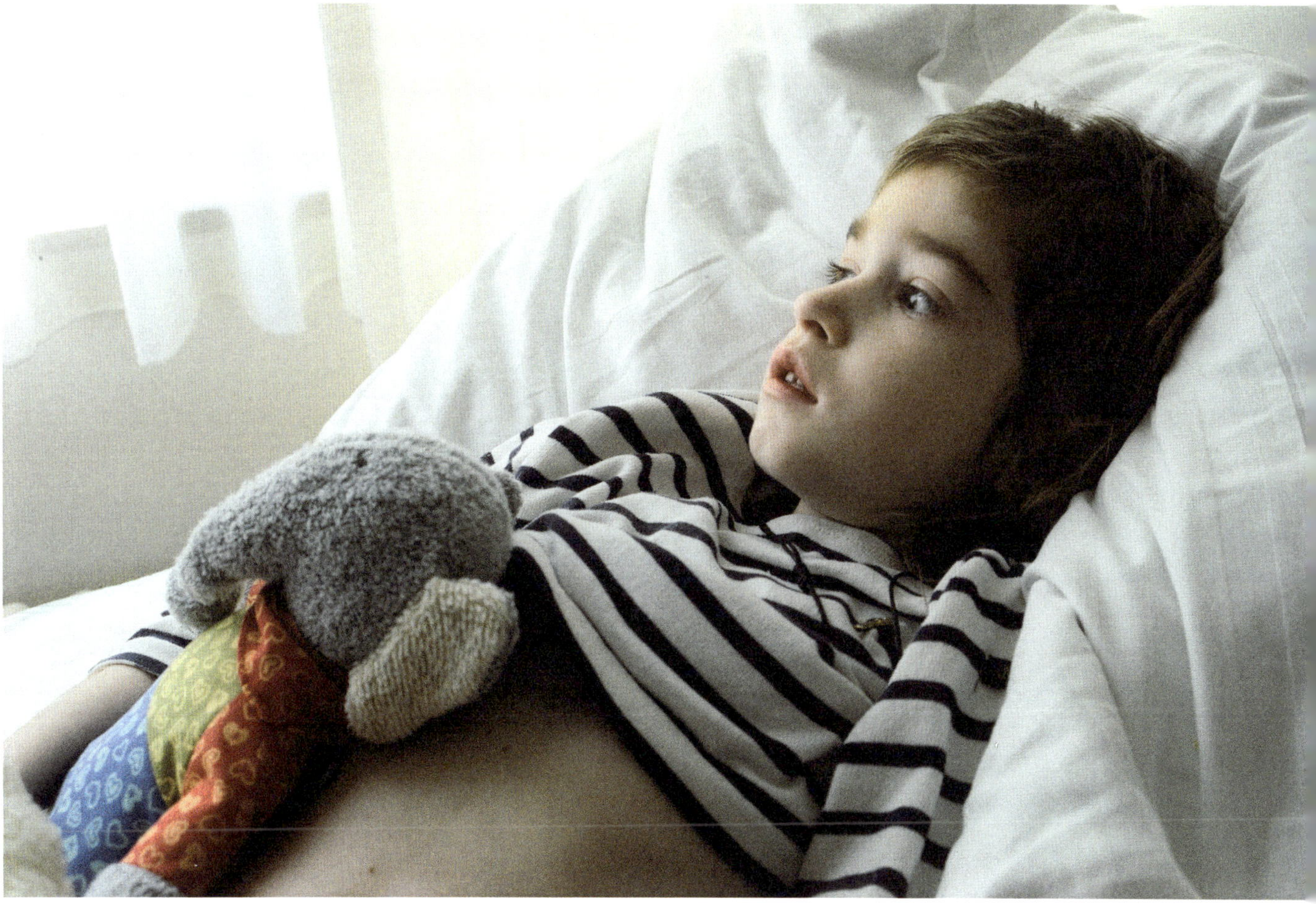

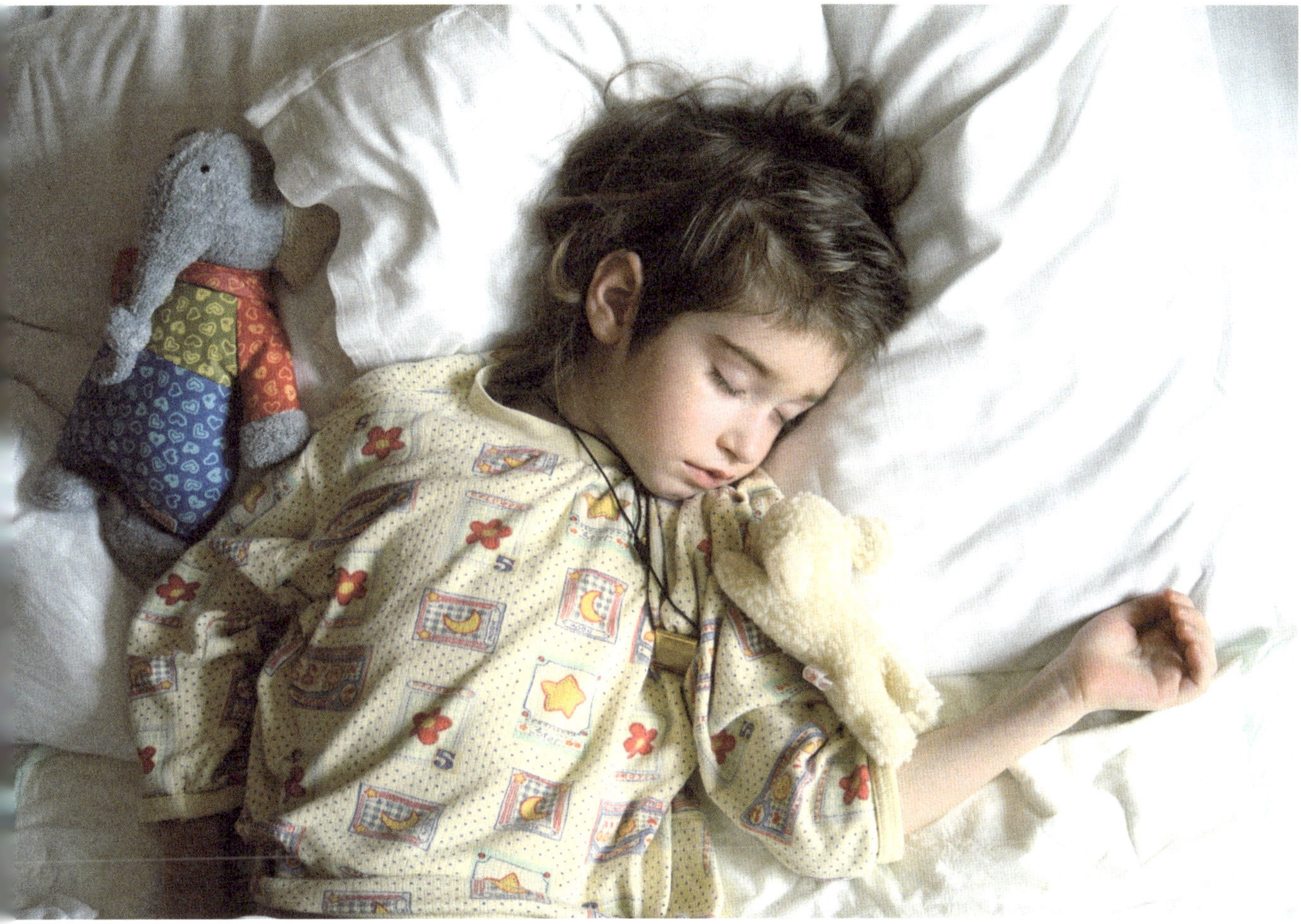

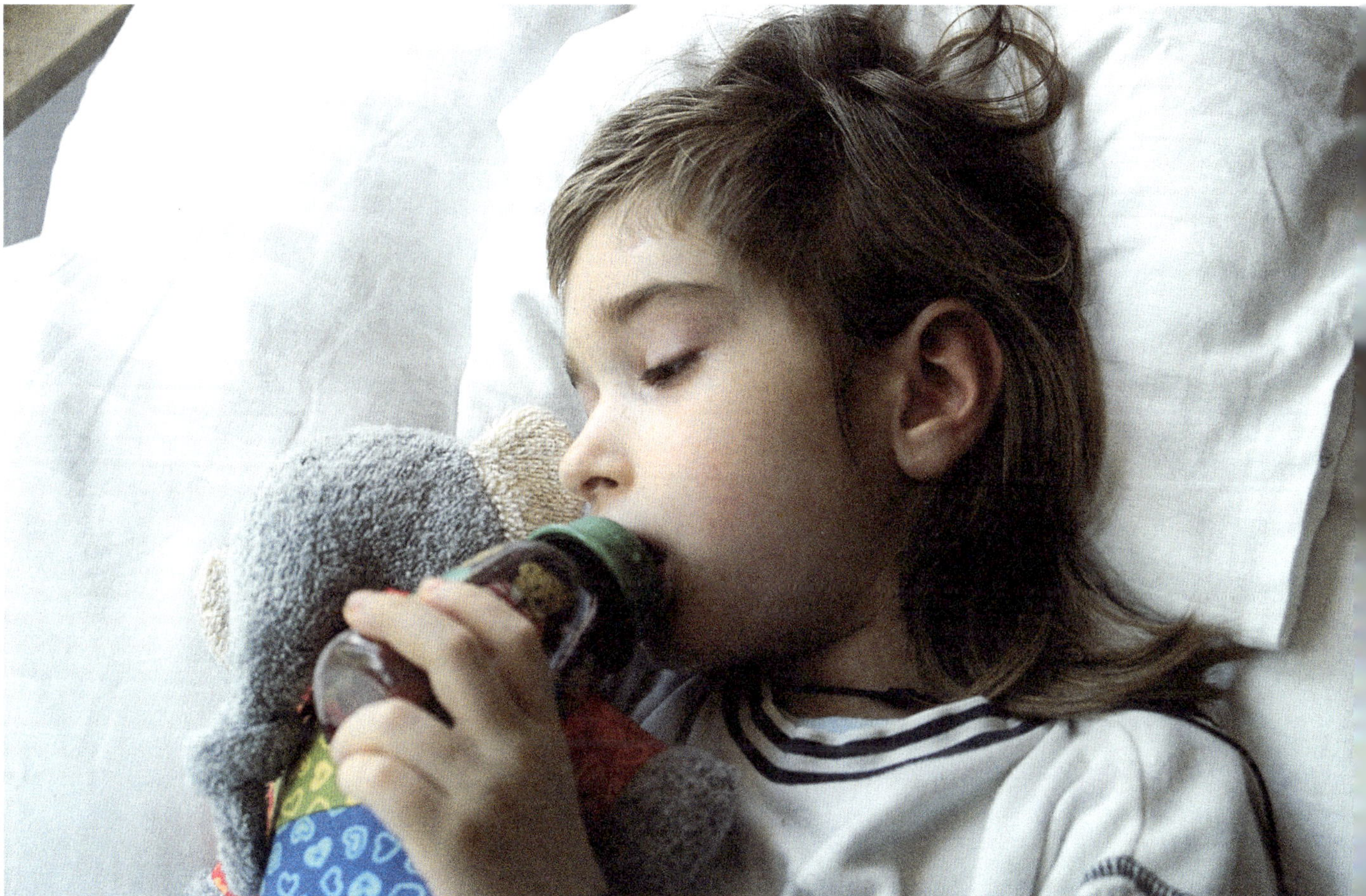

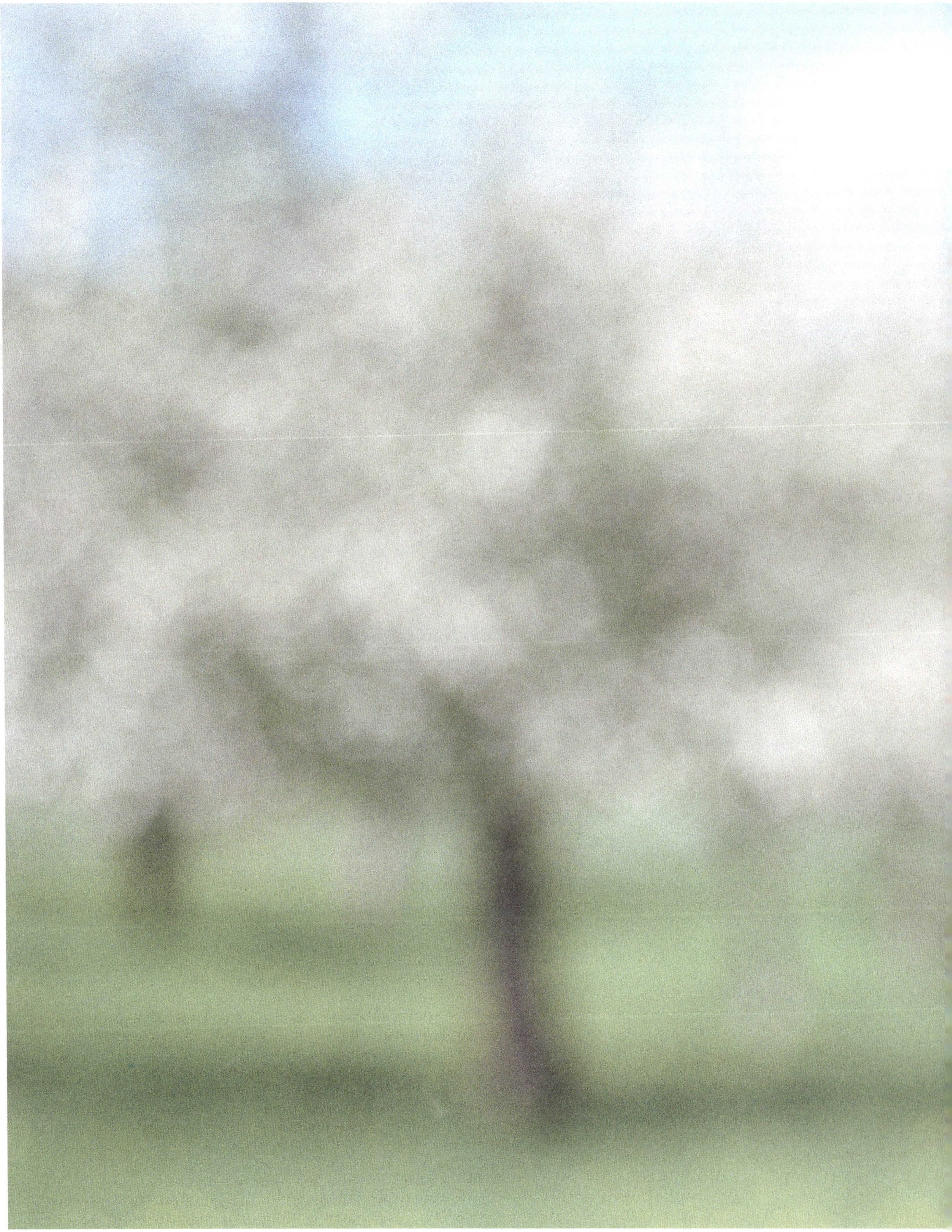

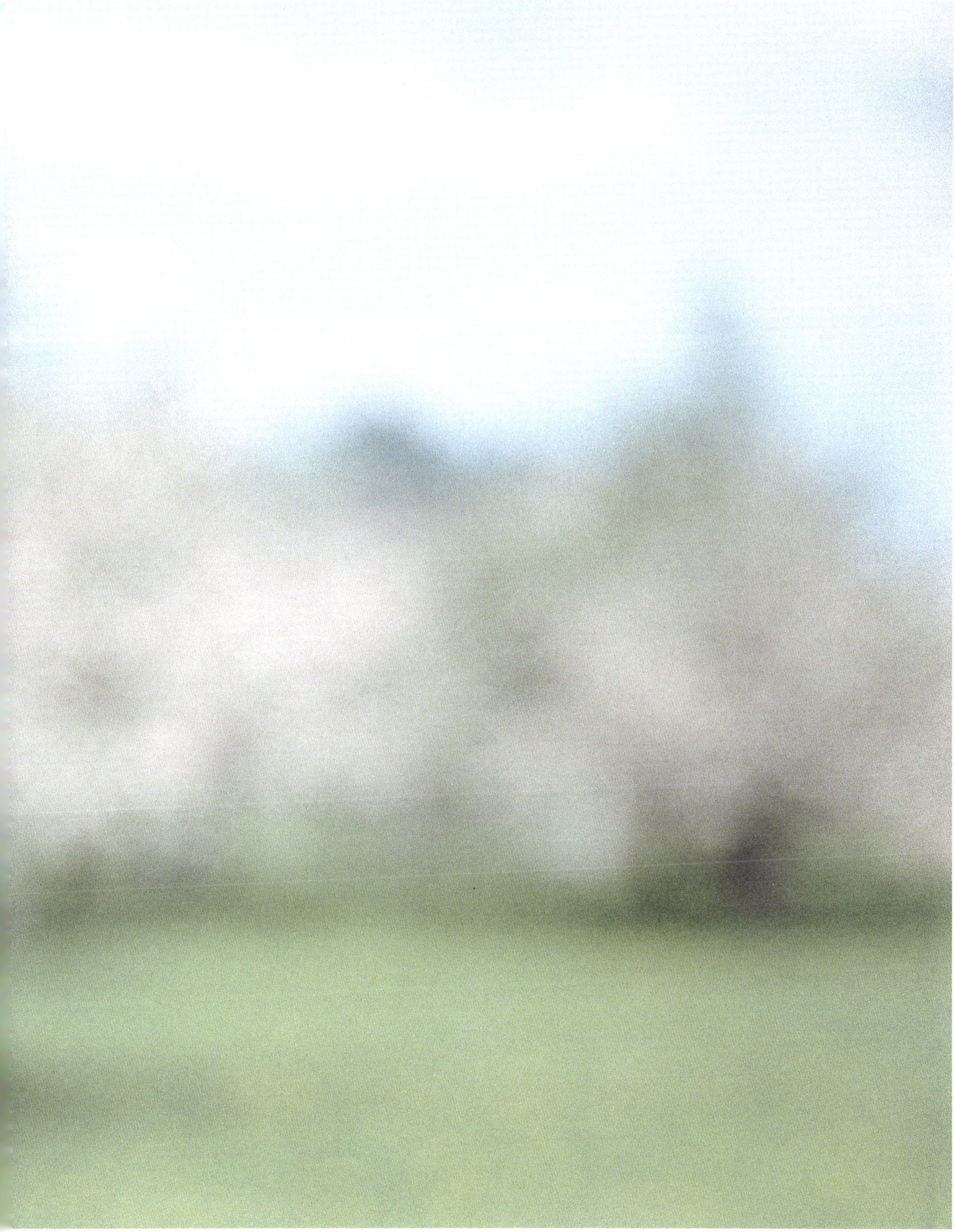

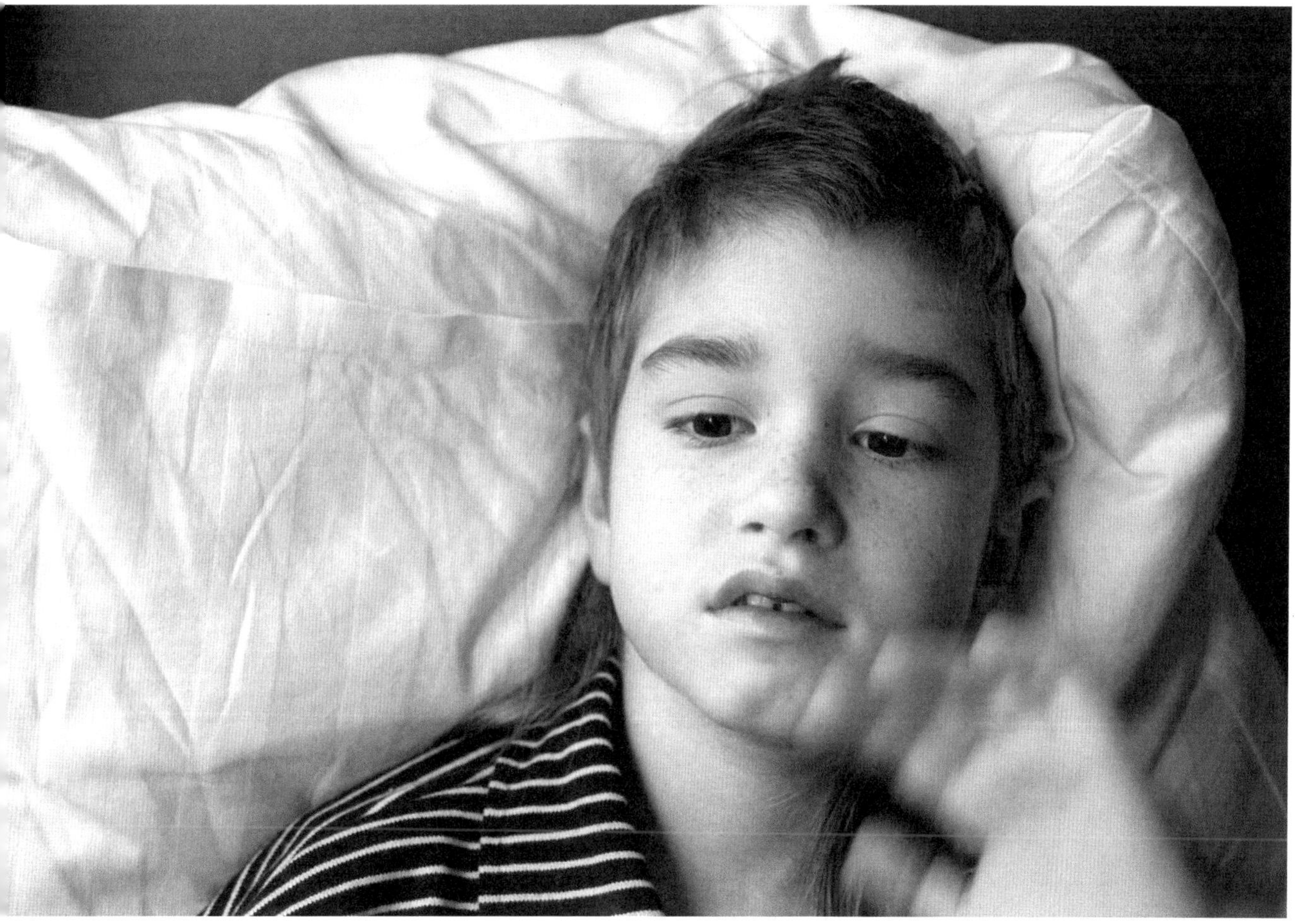

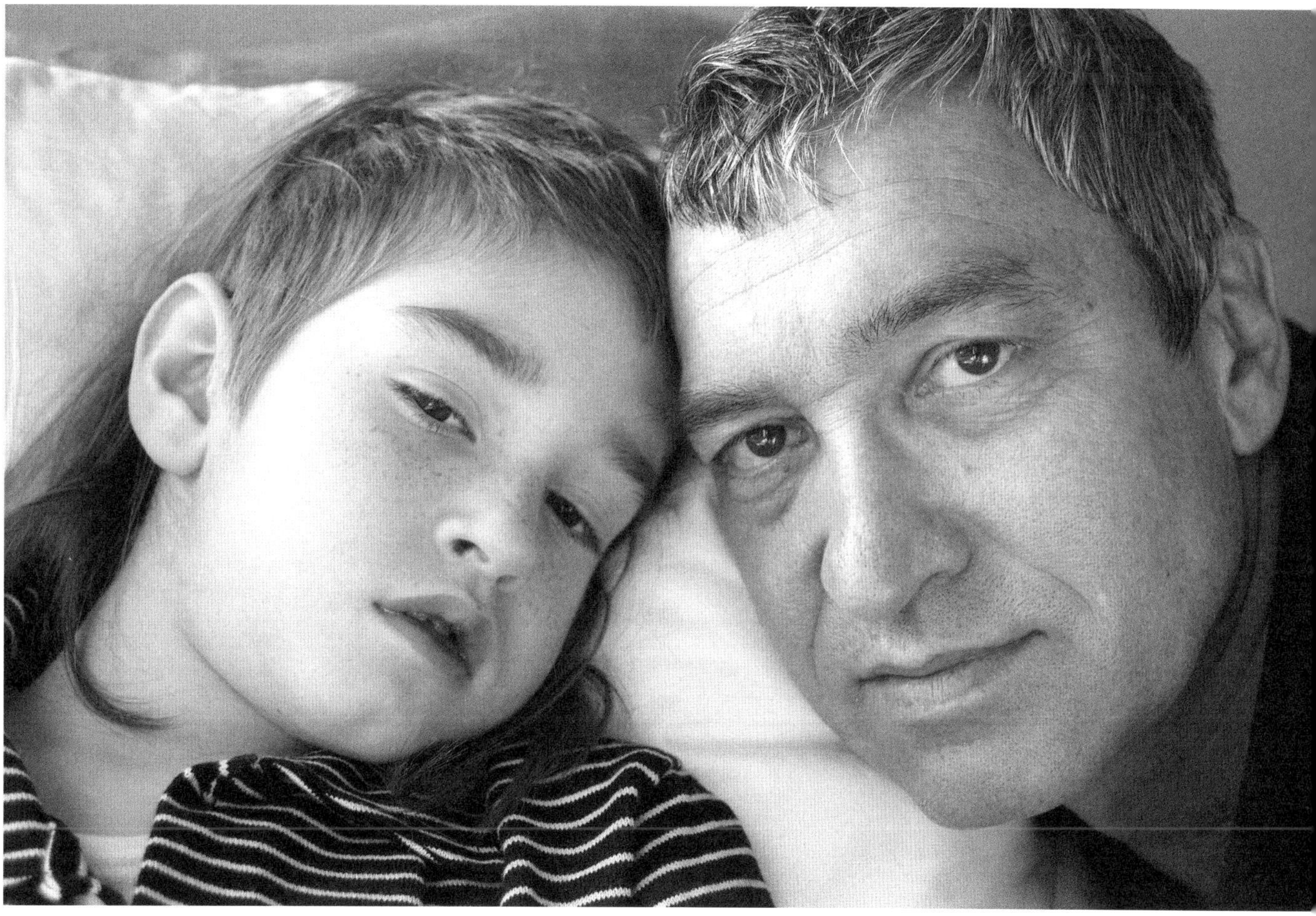

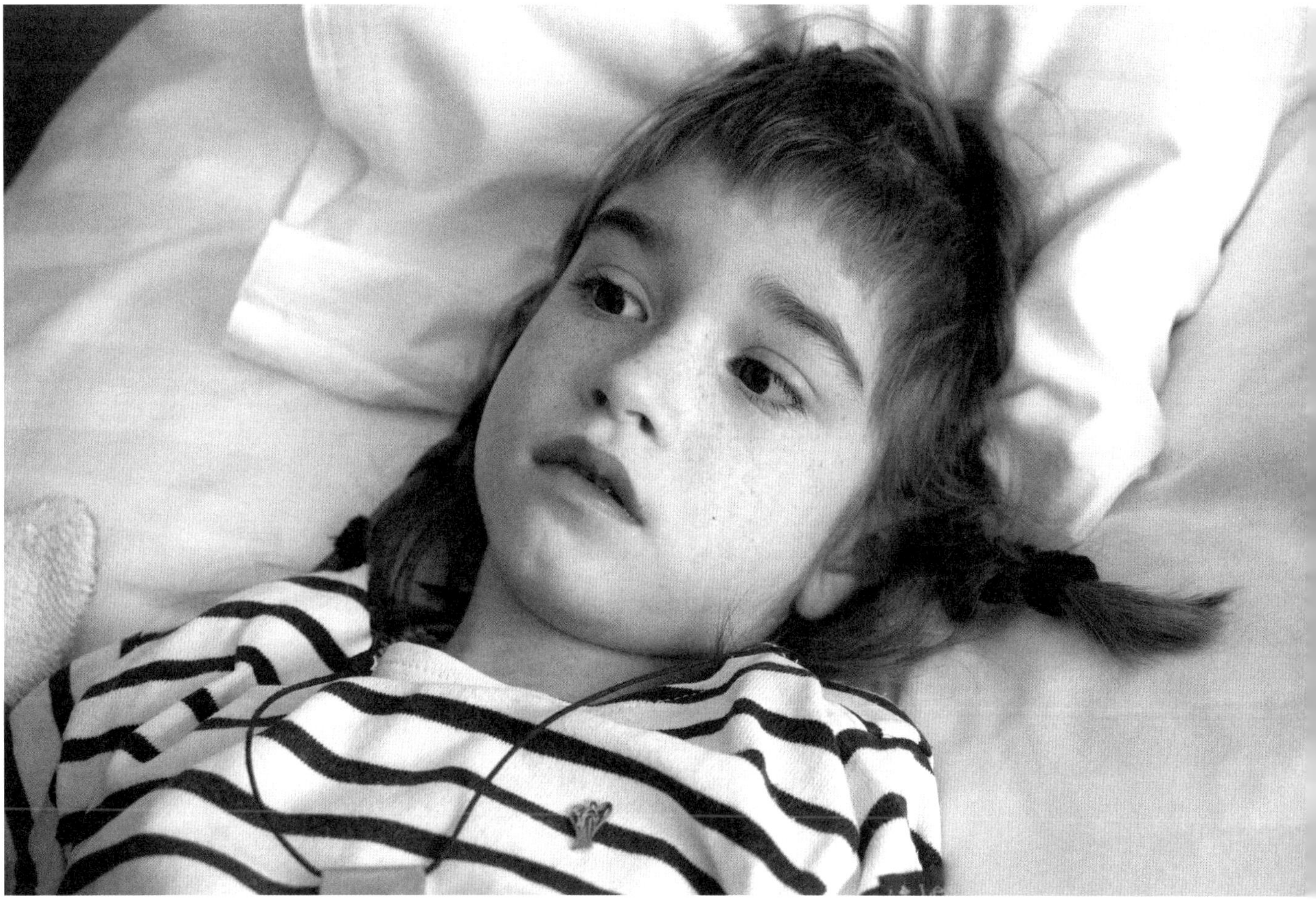

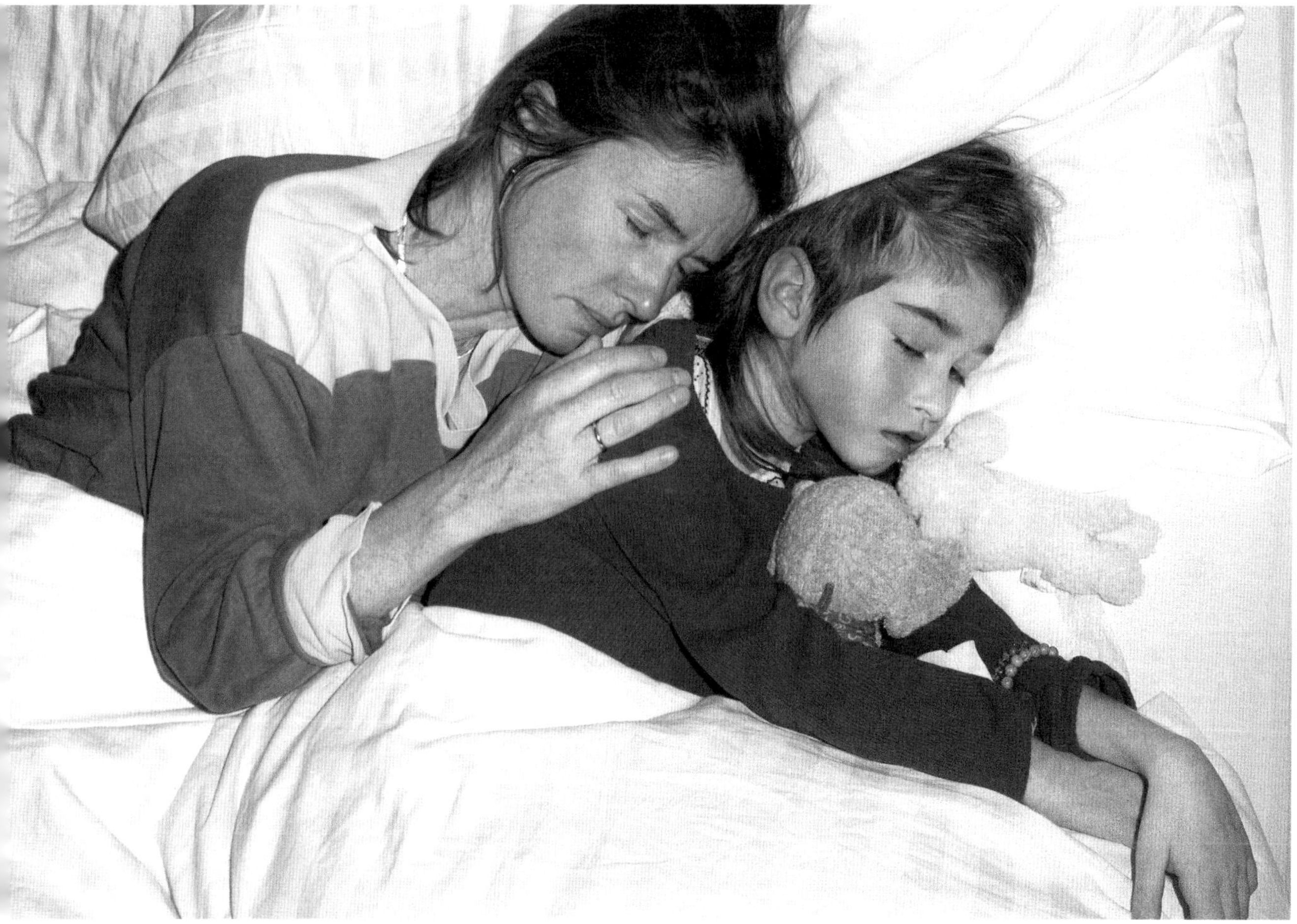

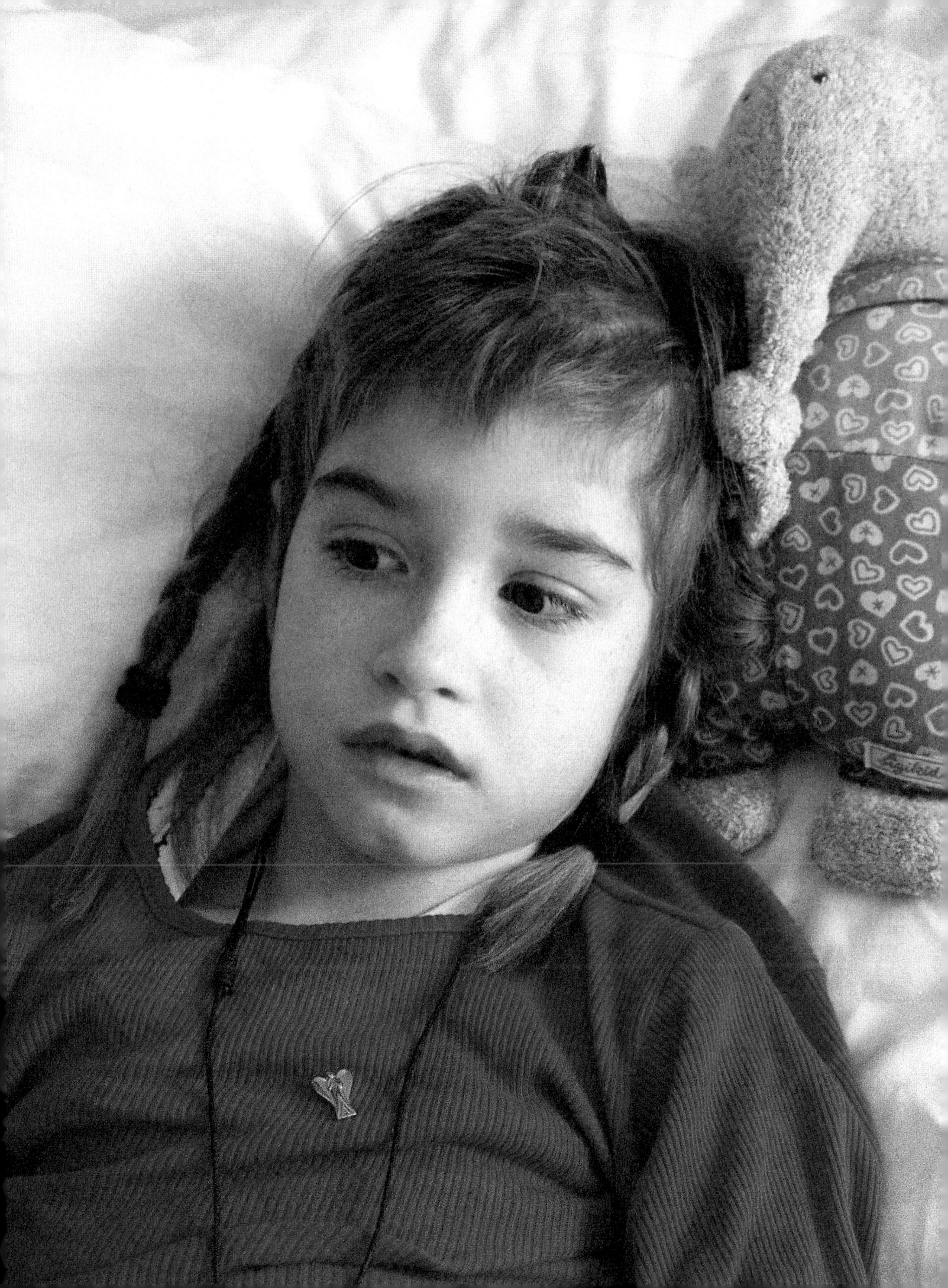

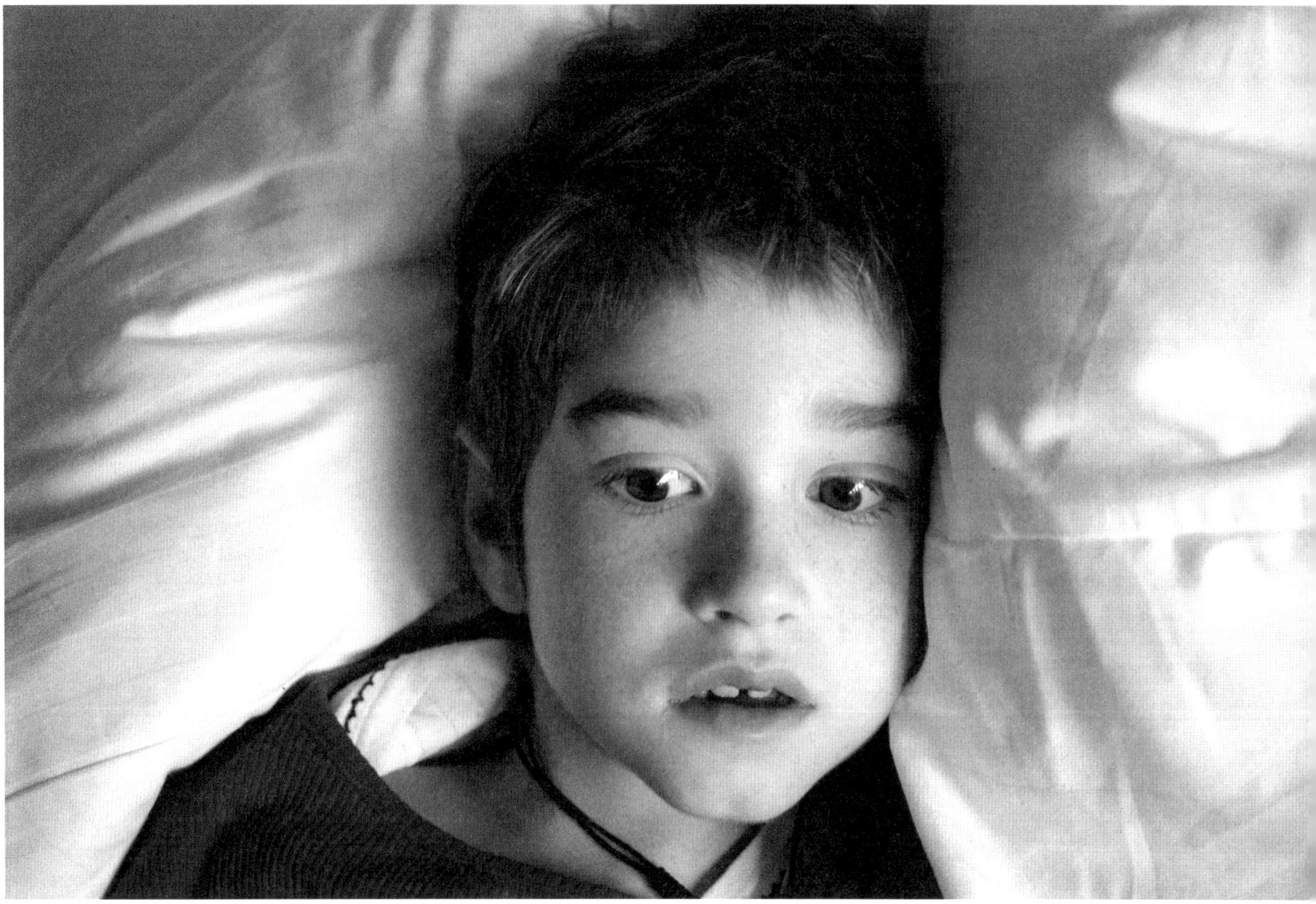

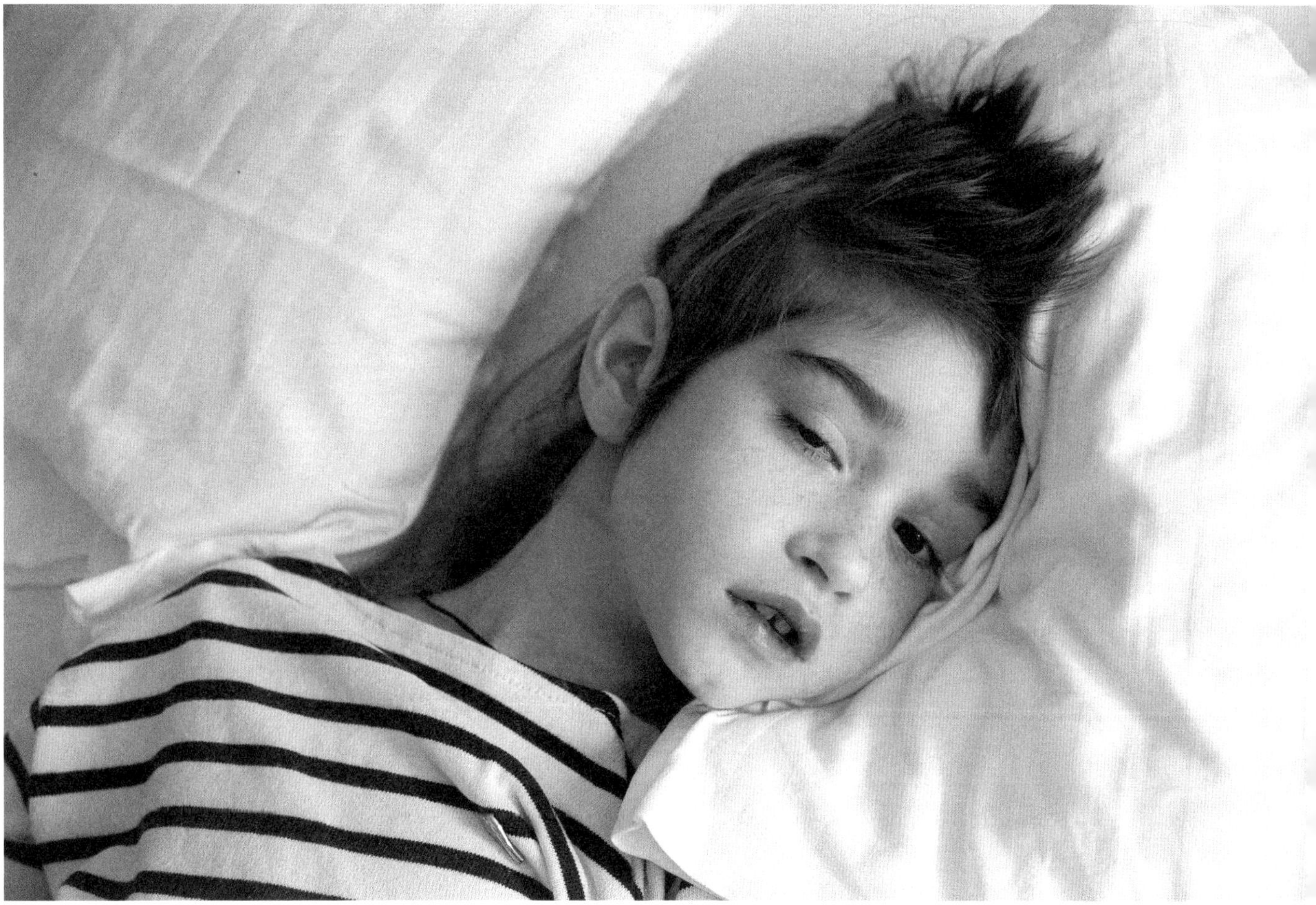

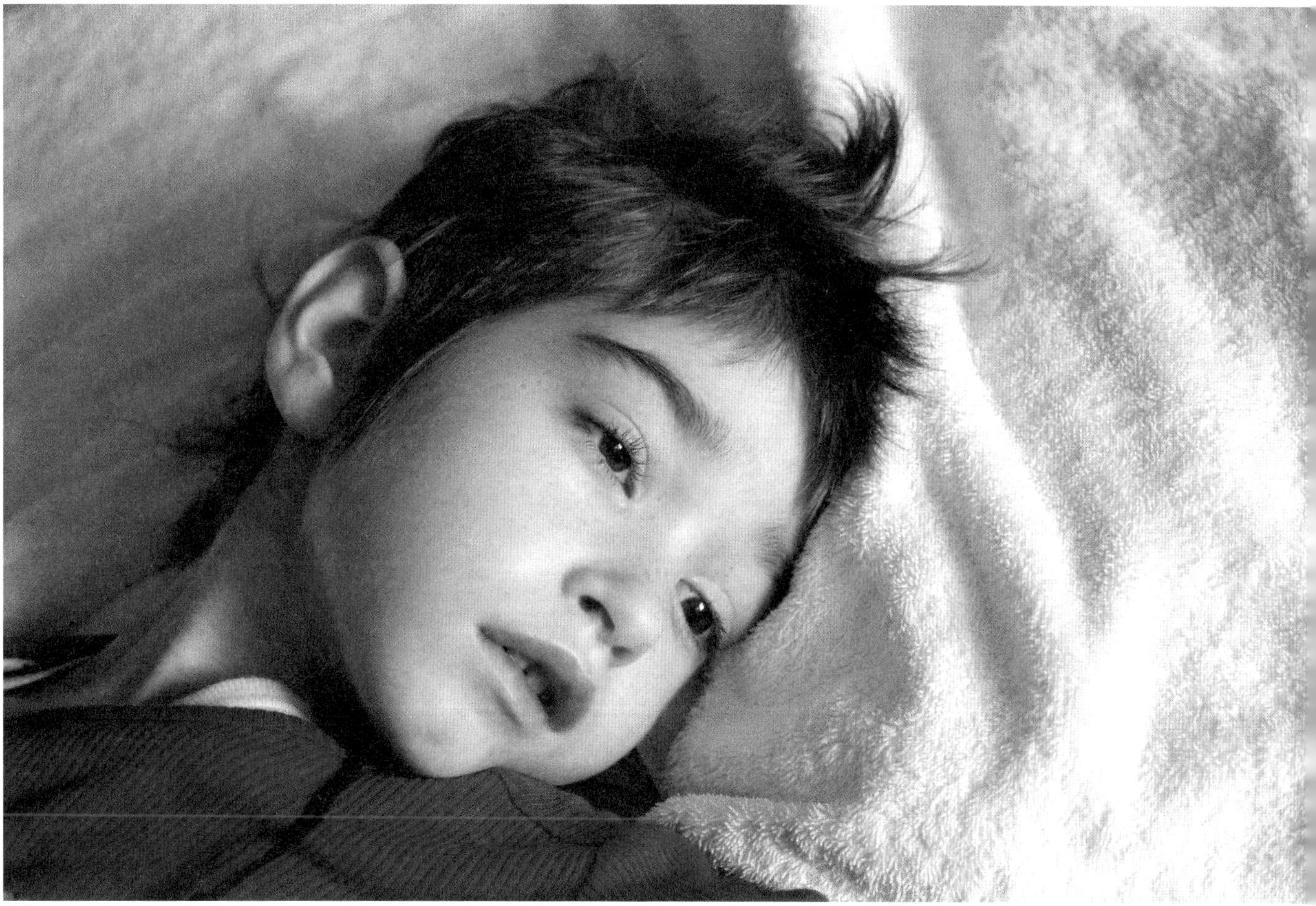

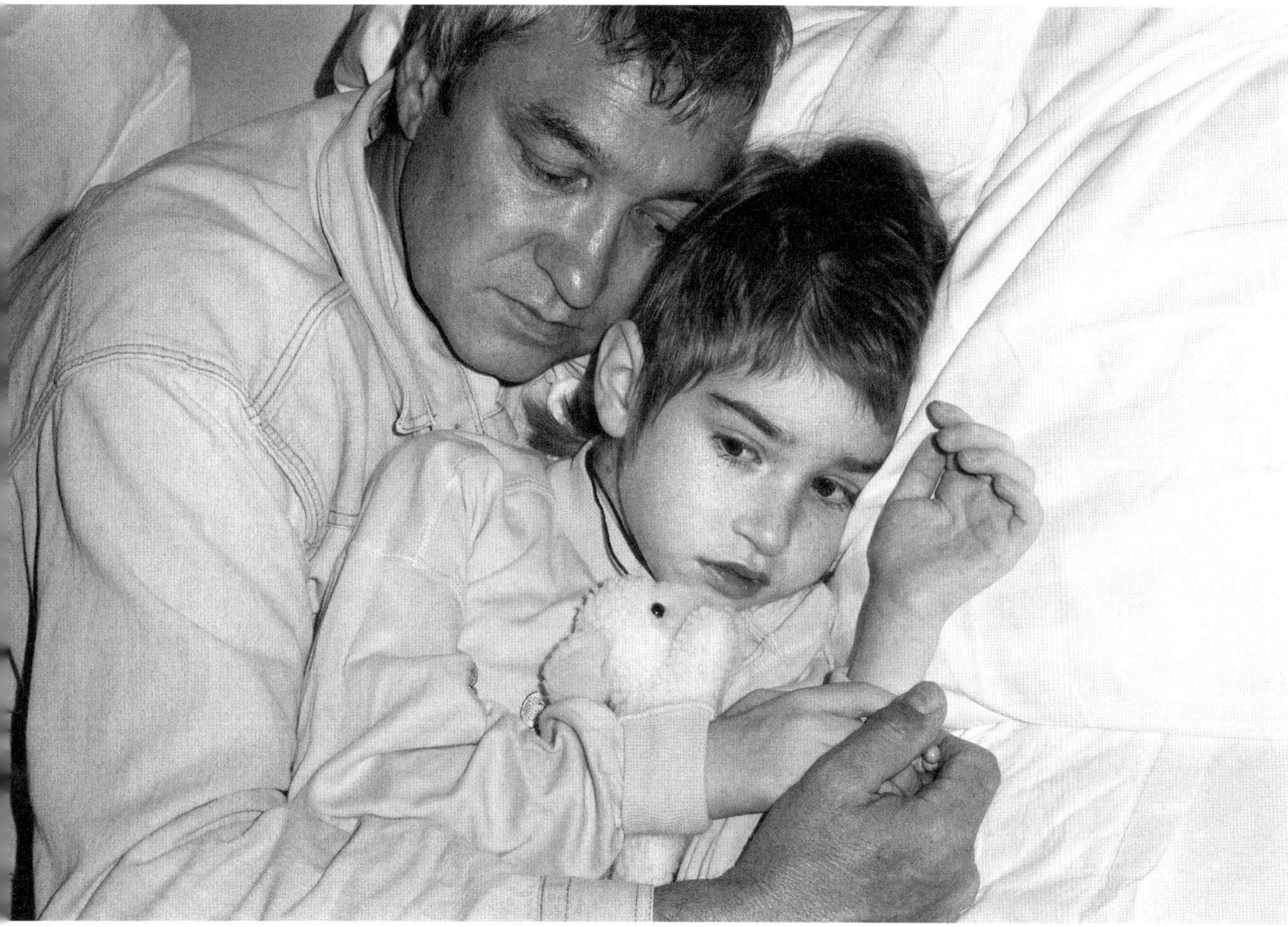

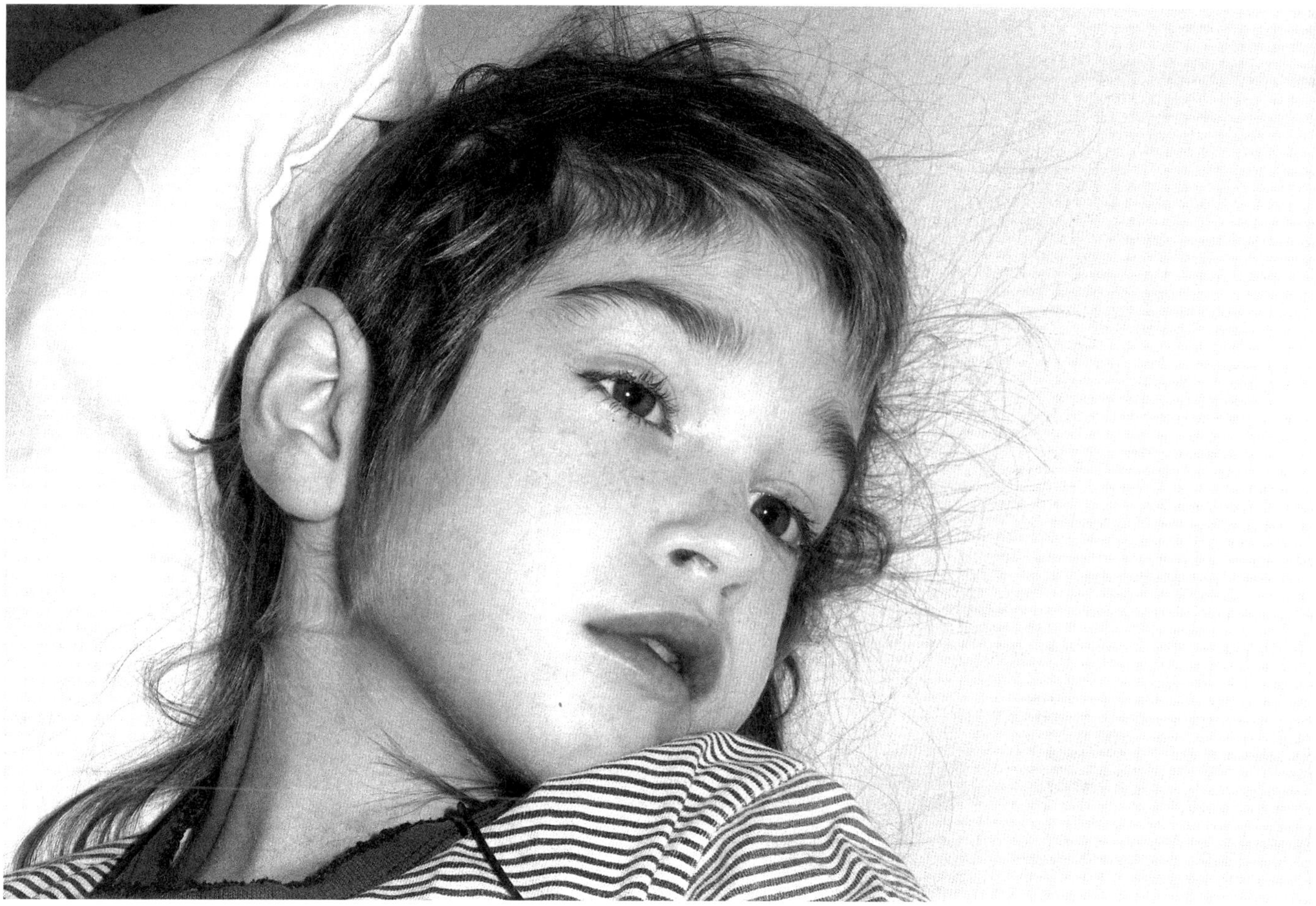

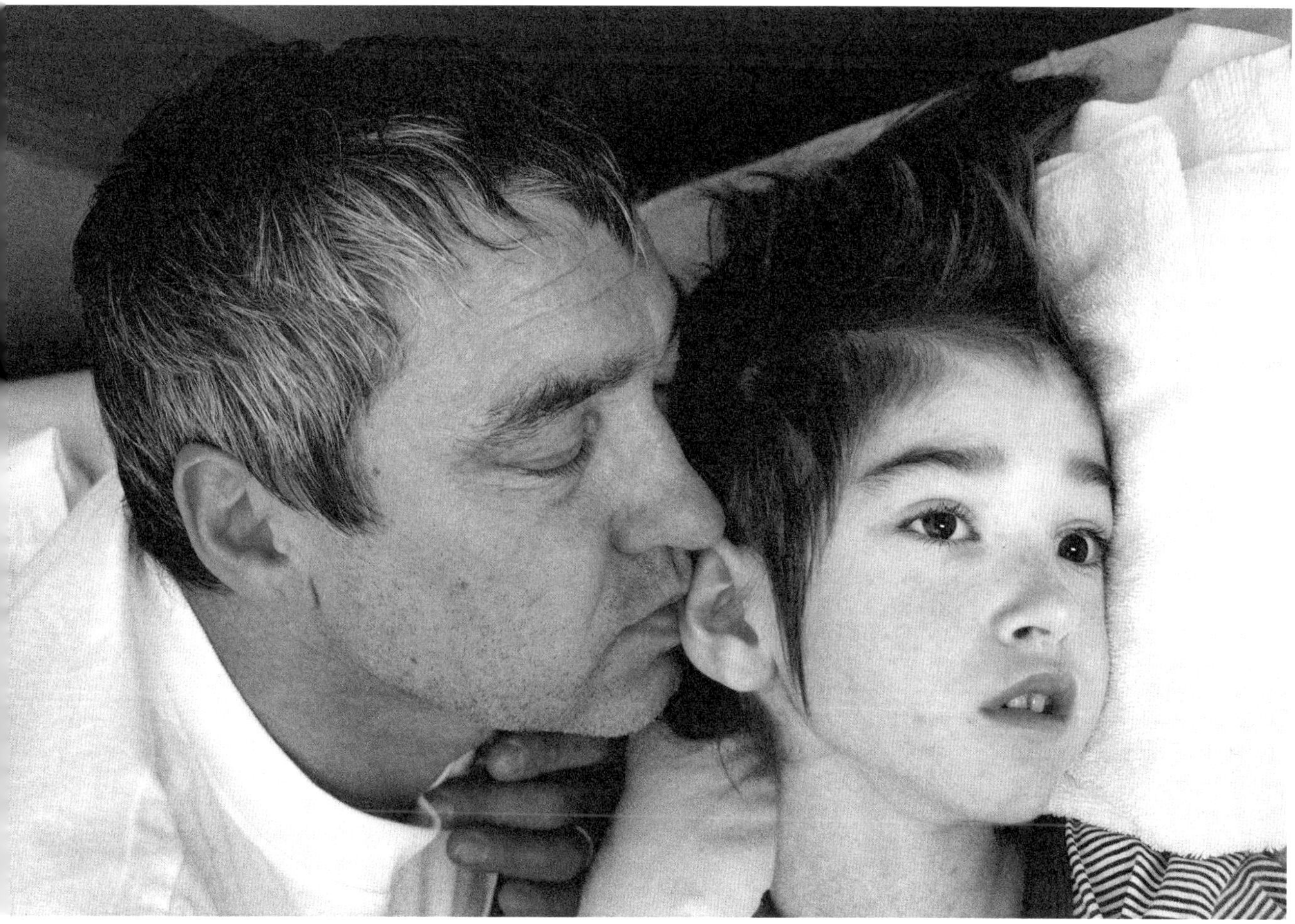

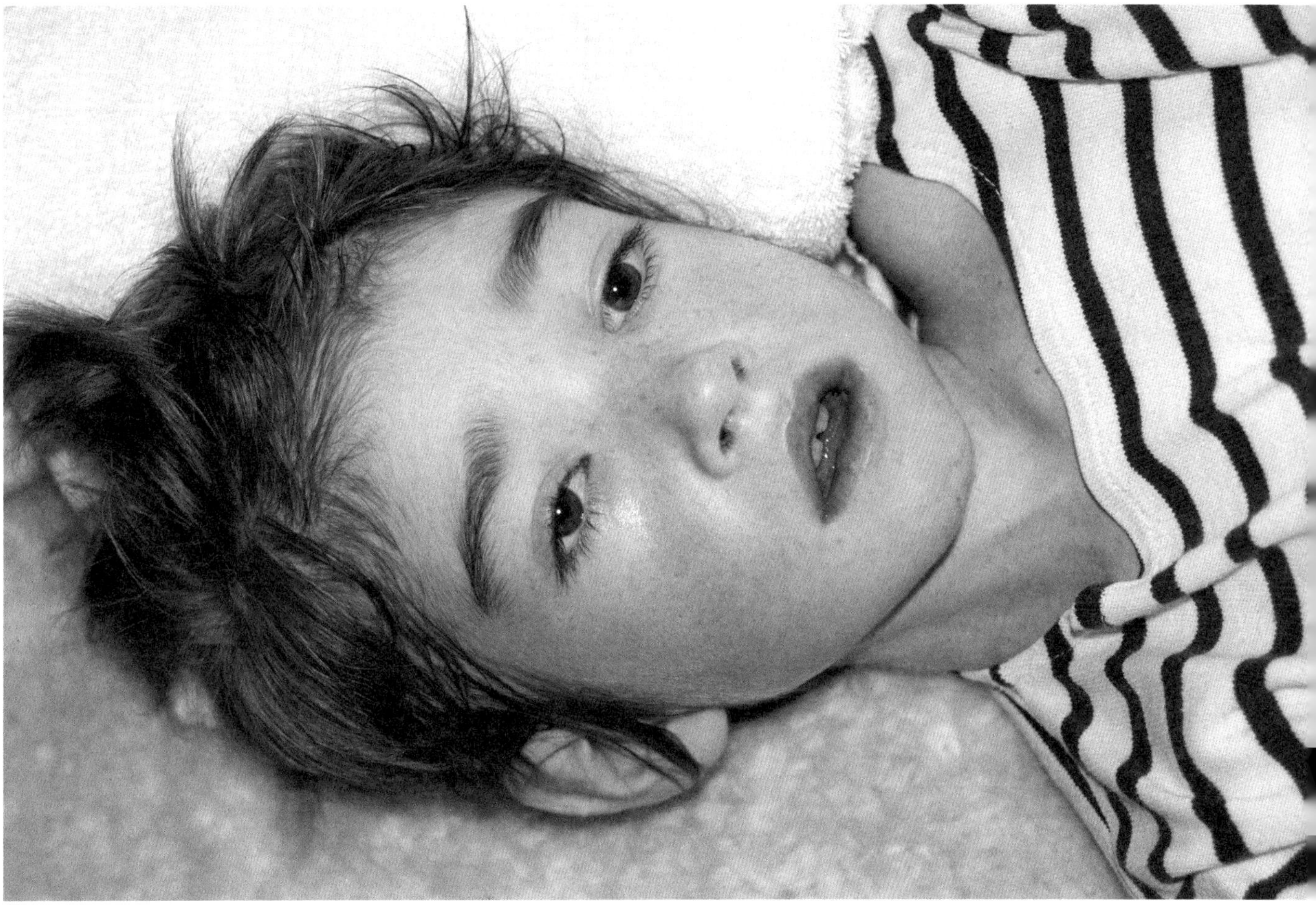

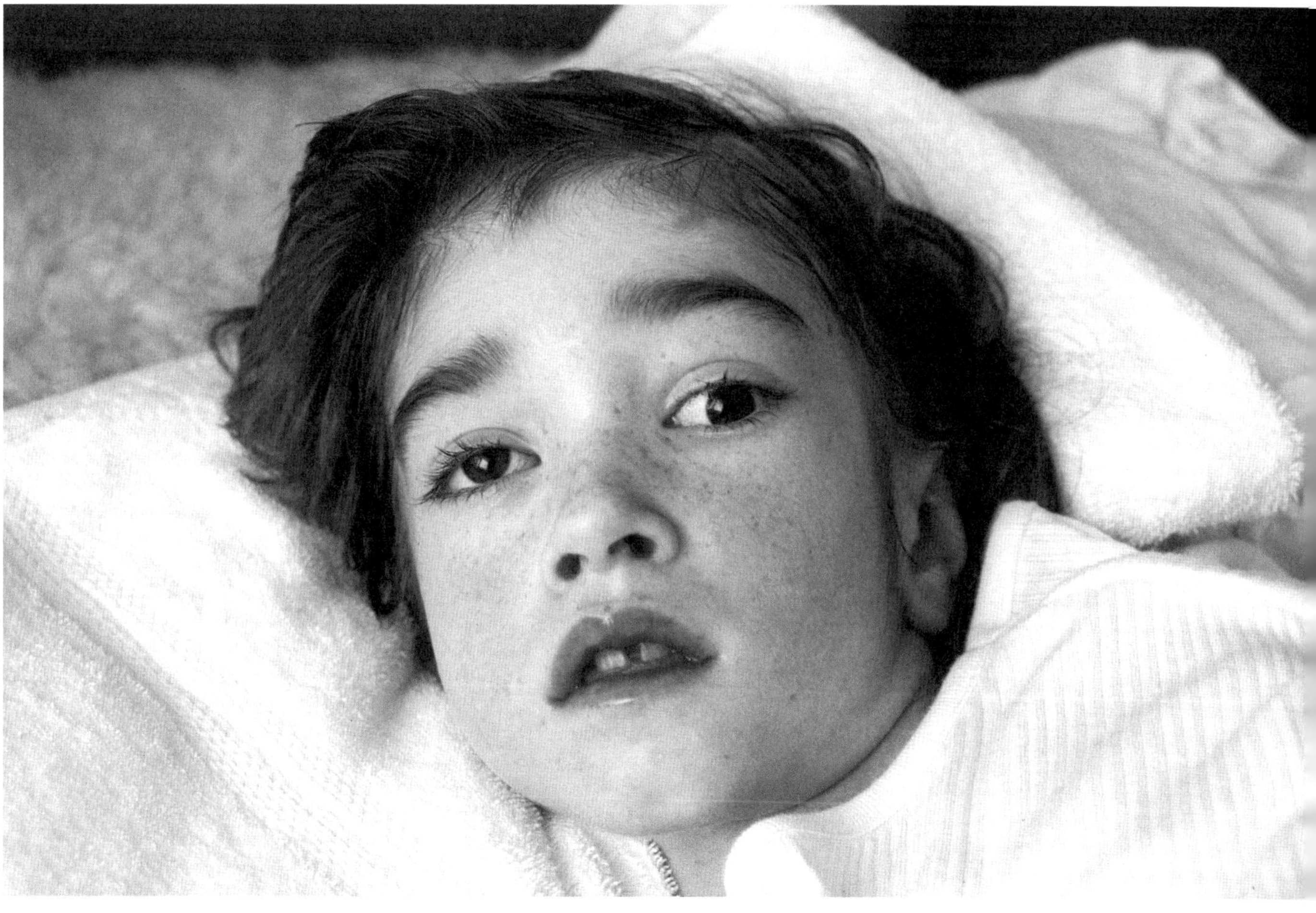

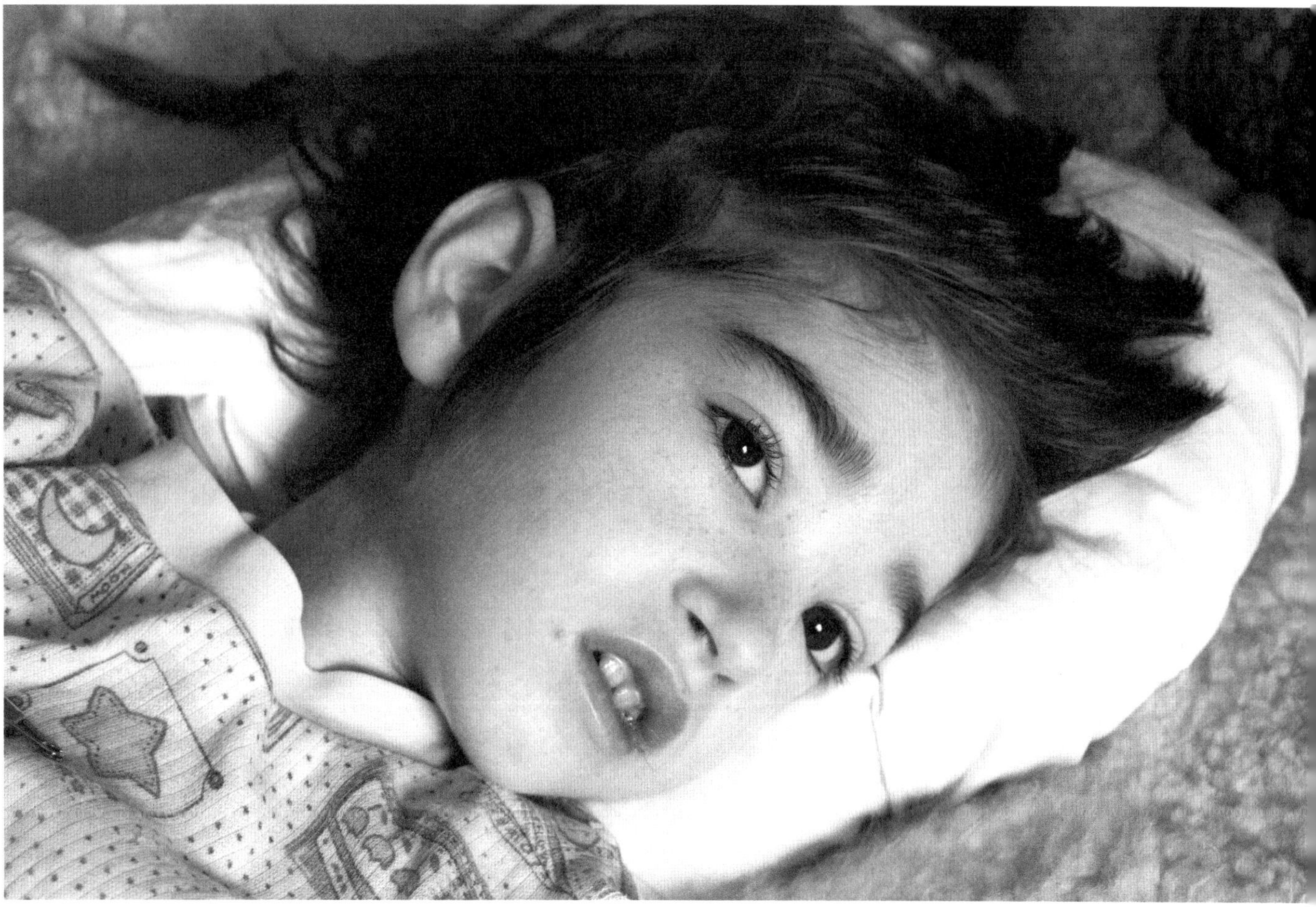

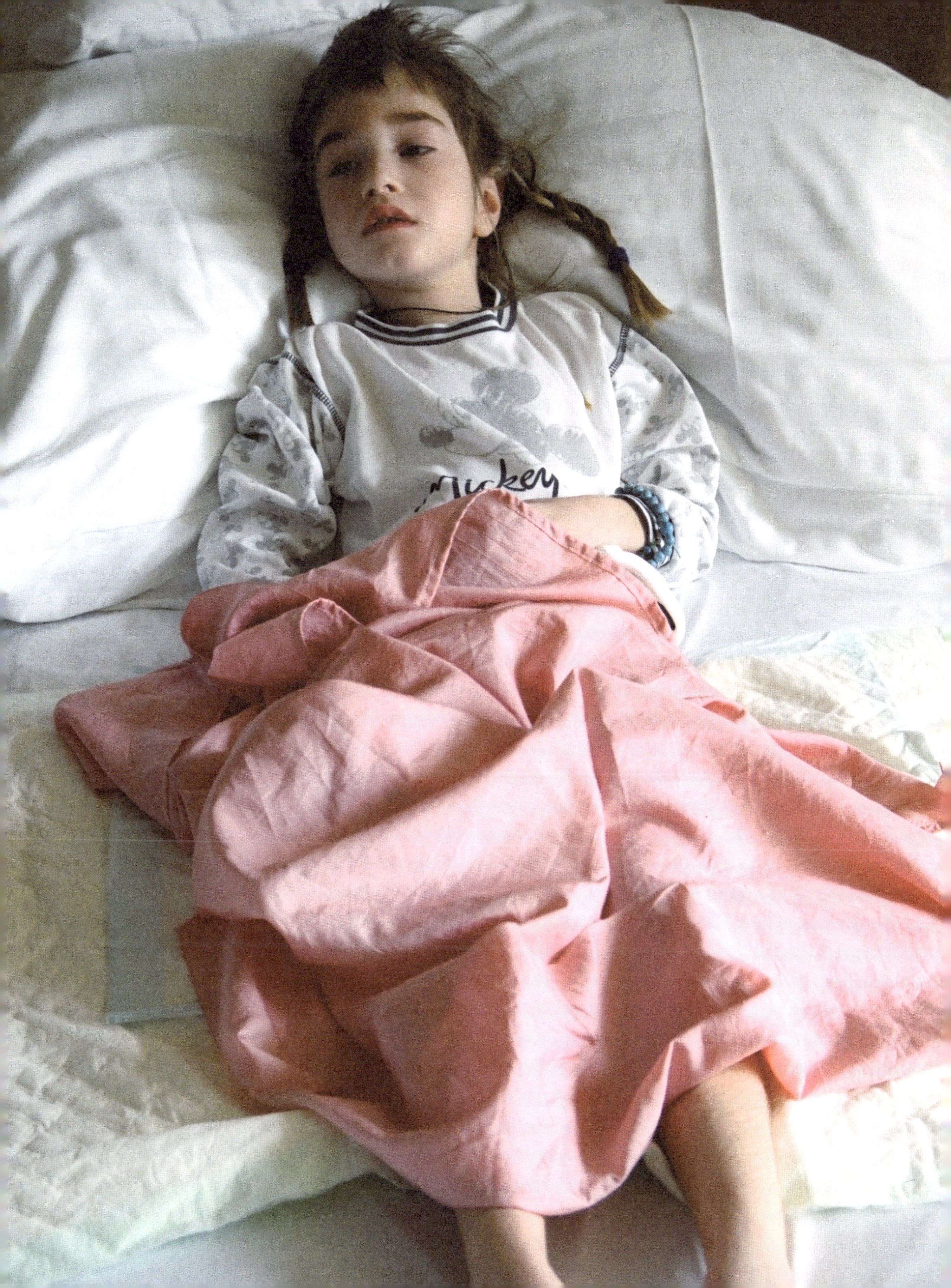
Mickey

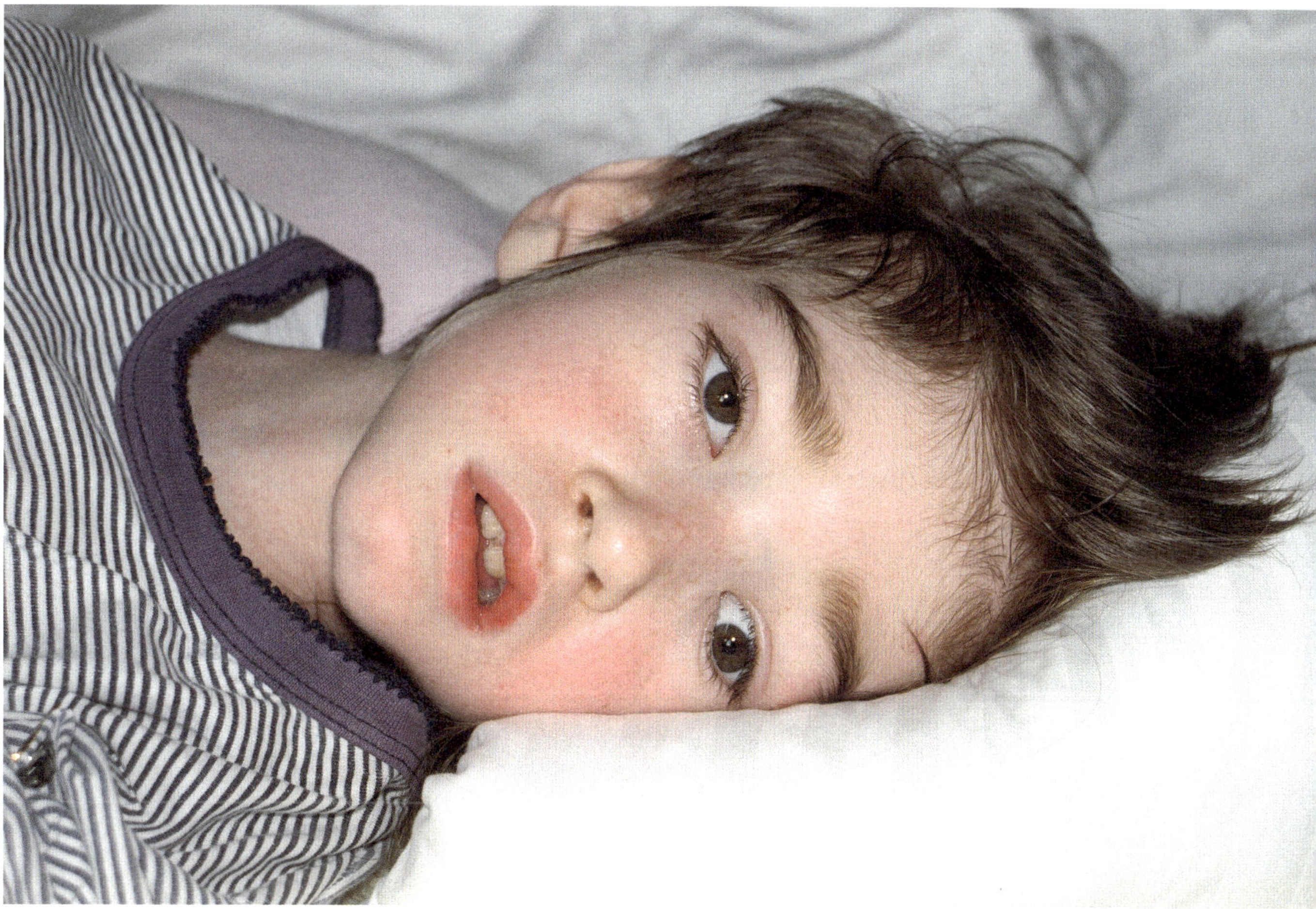

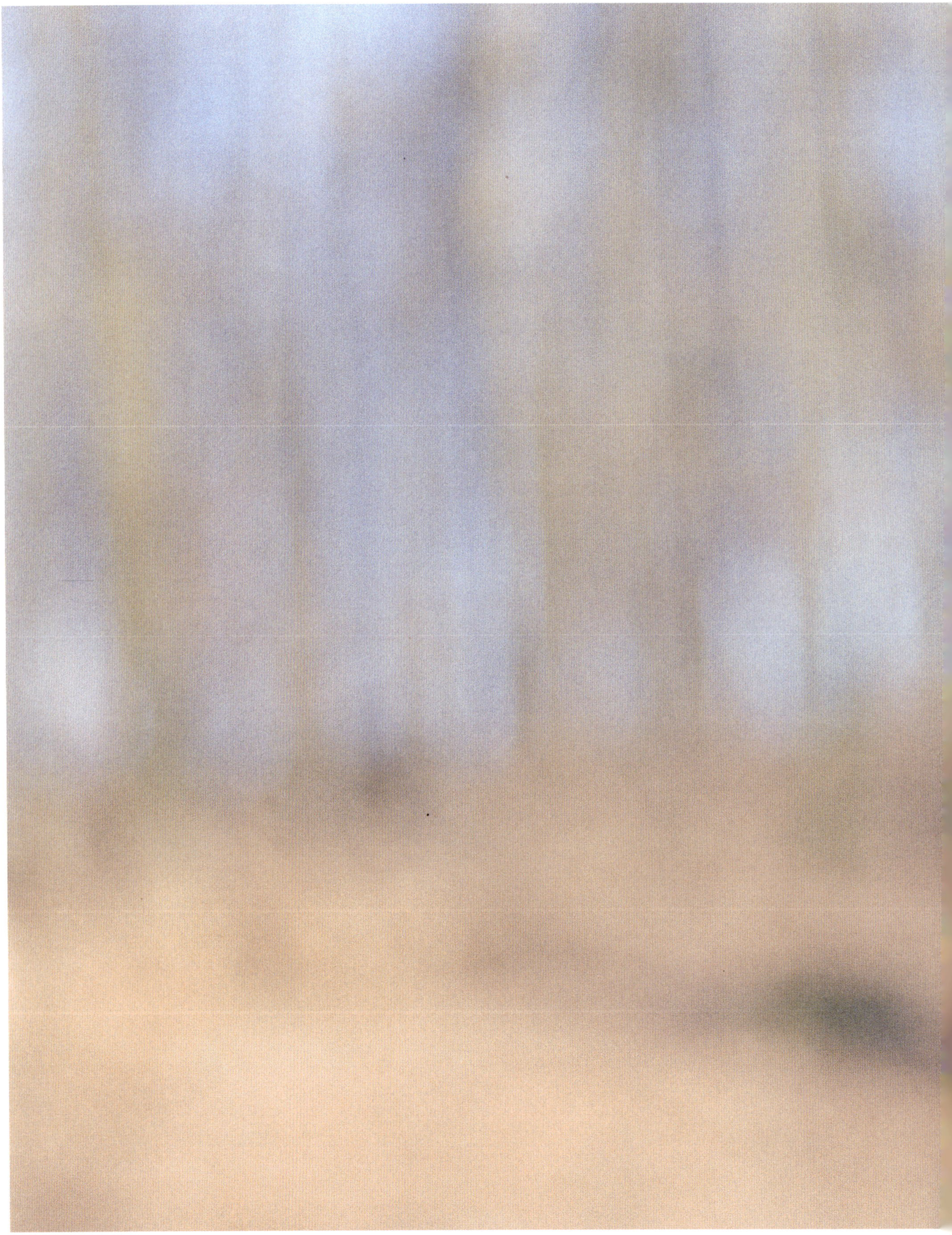

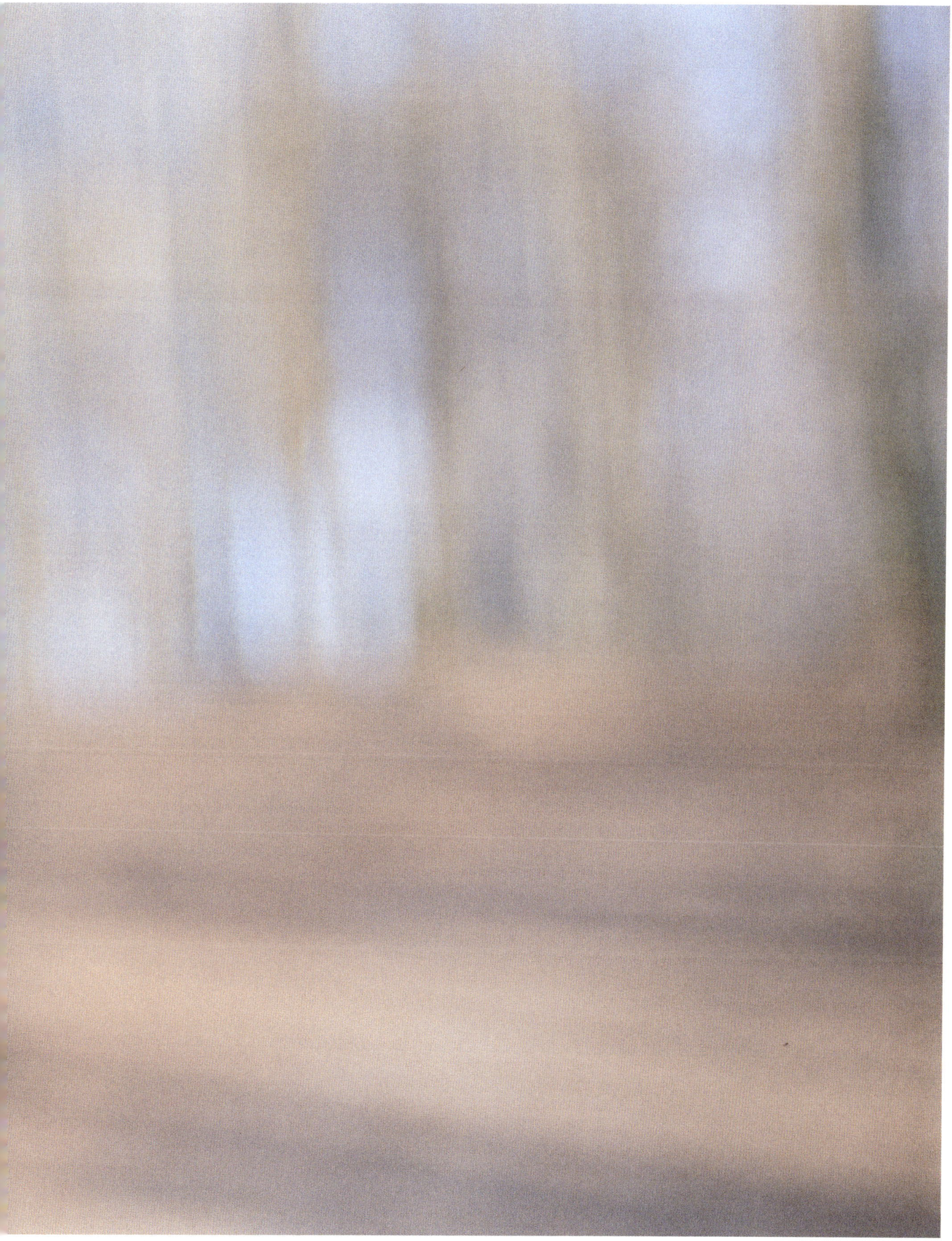

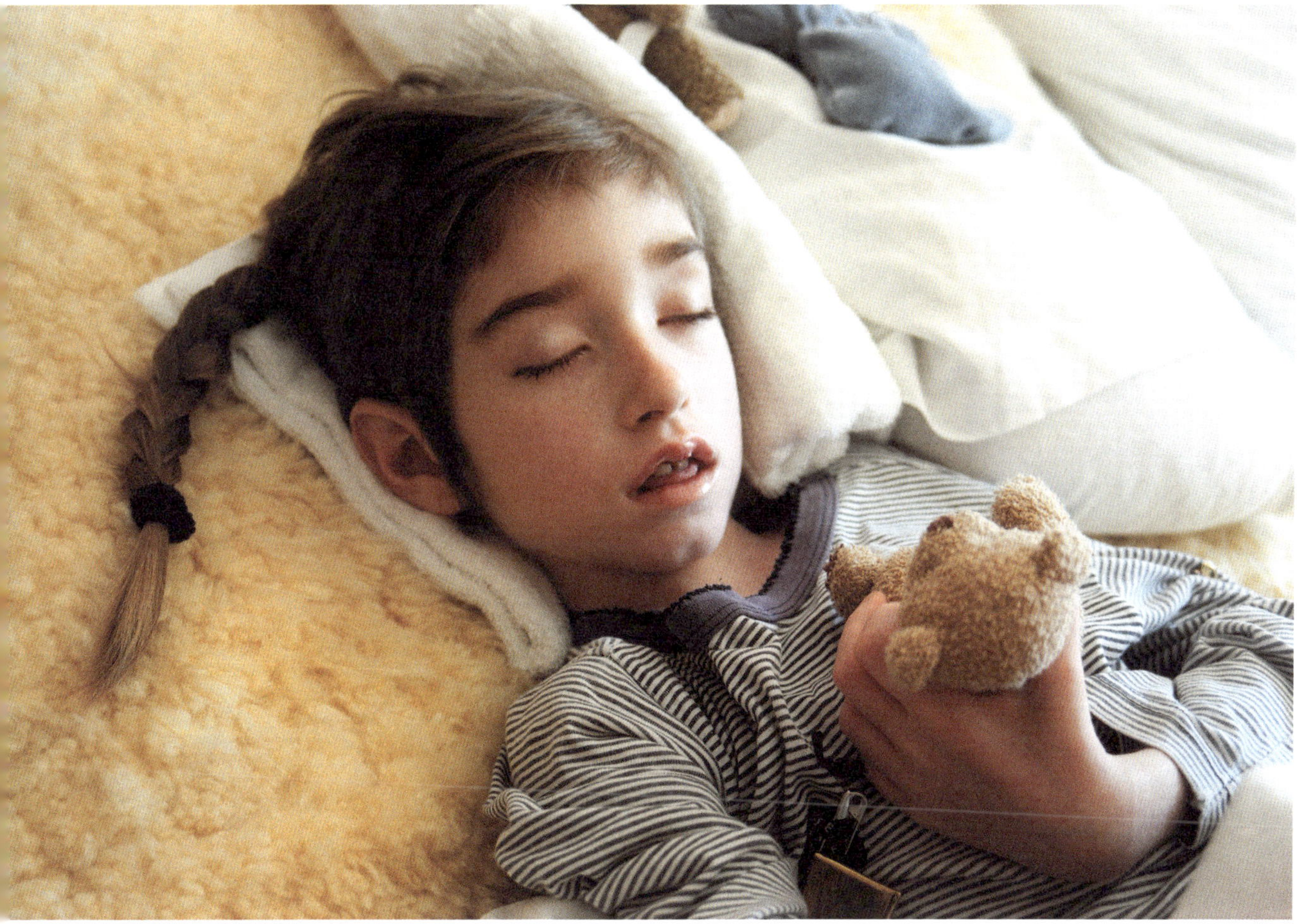

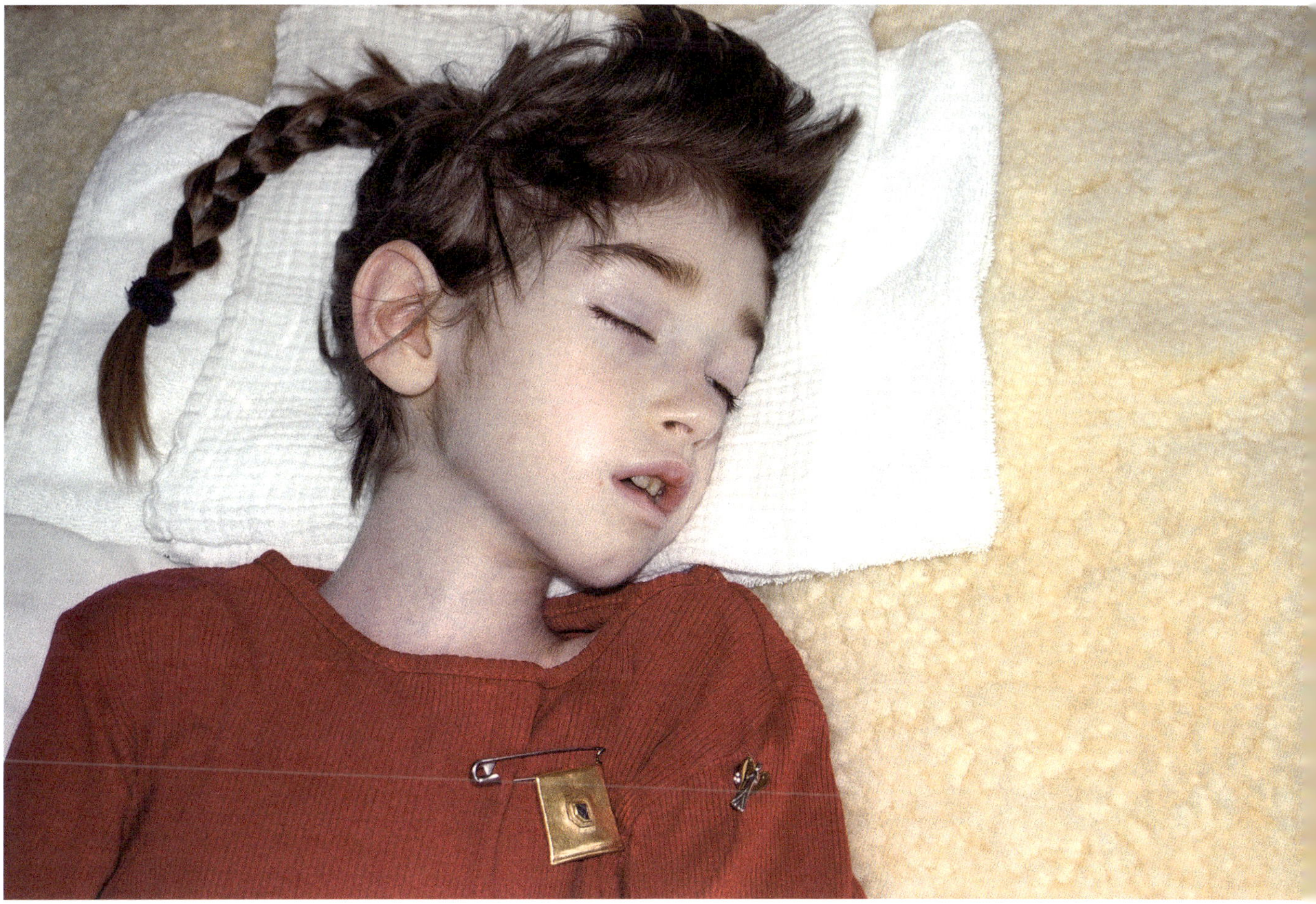

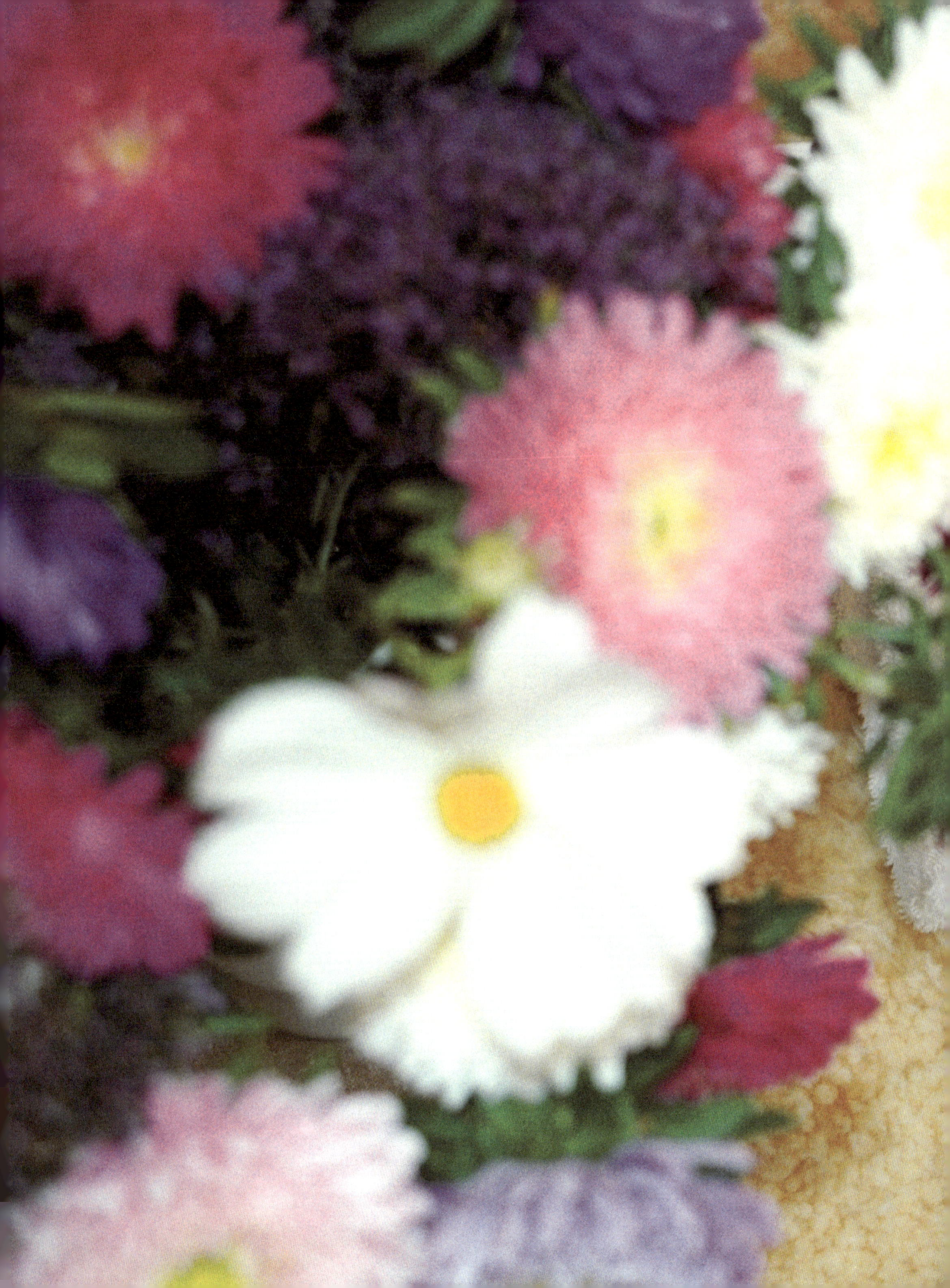

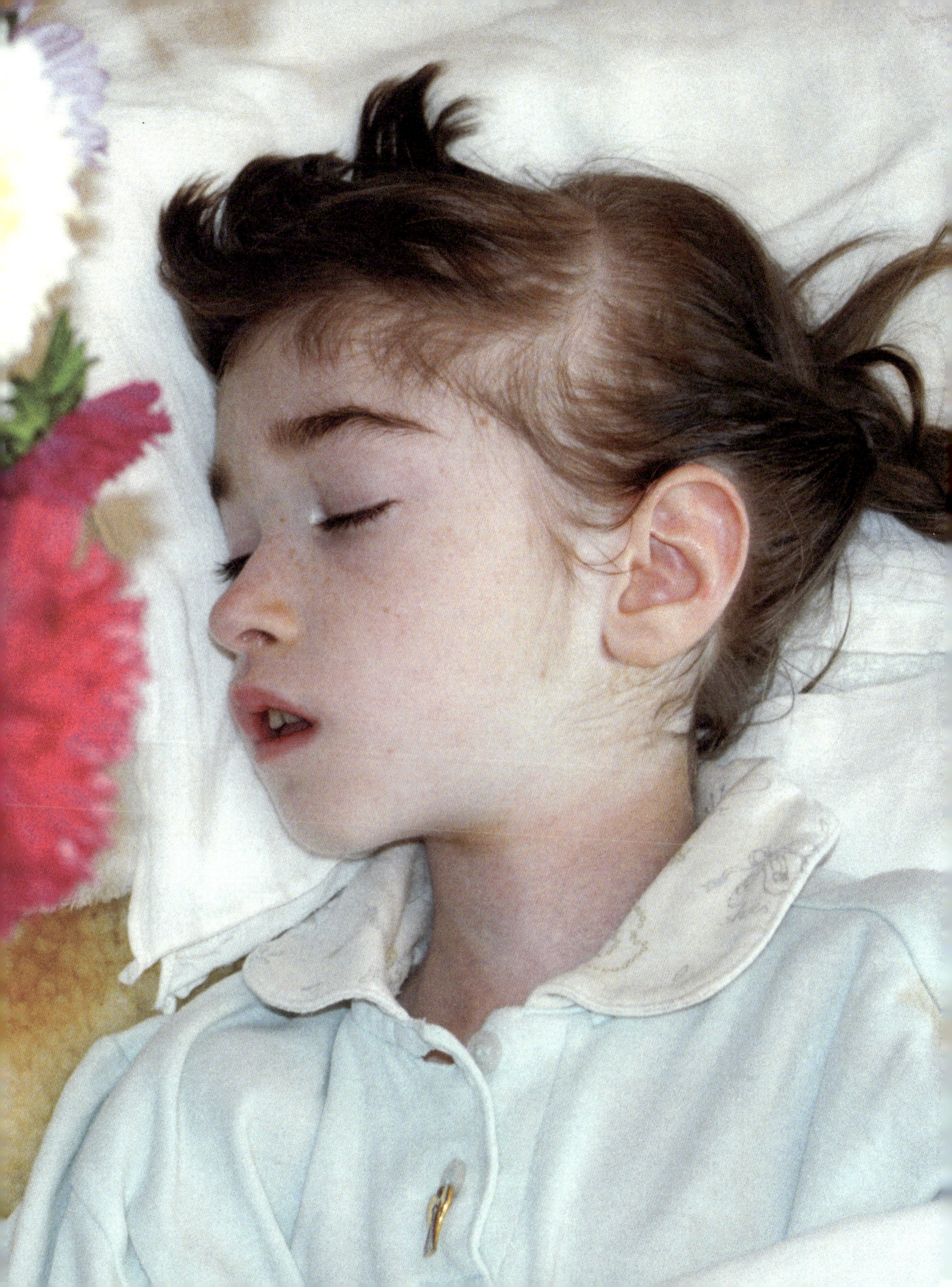

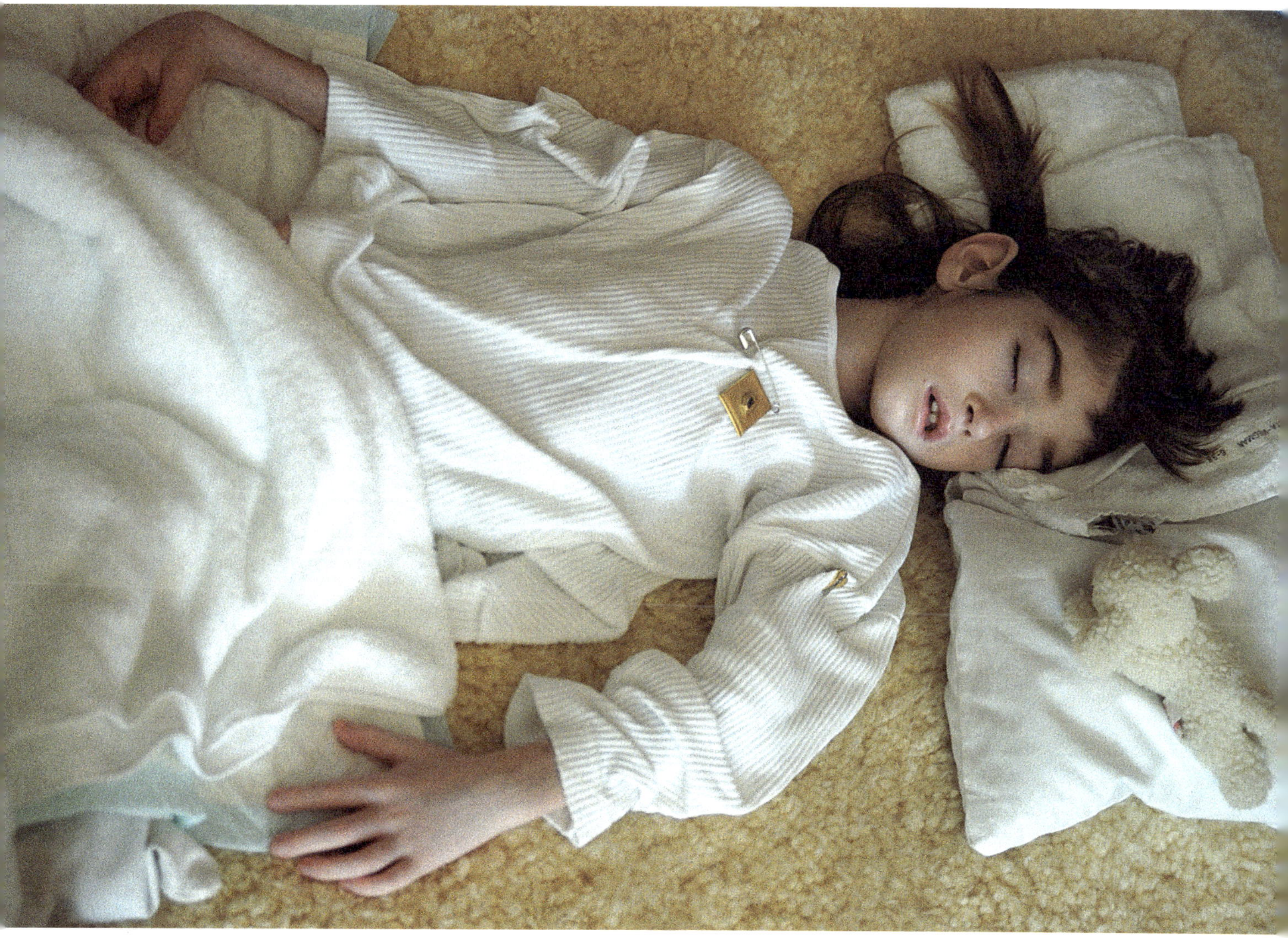

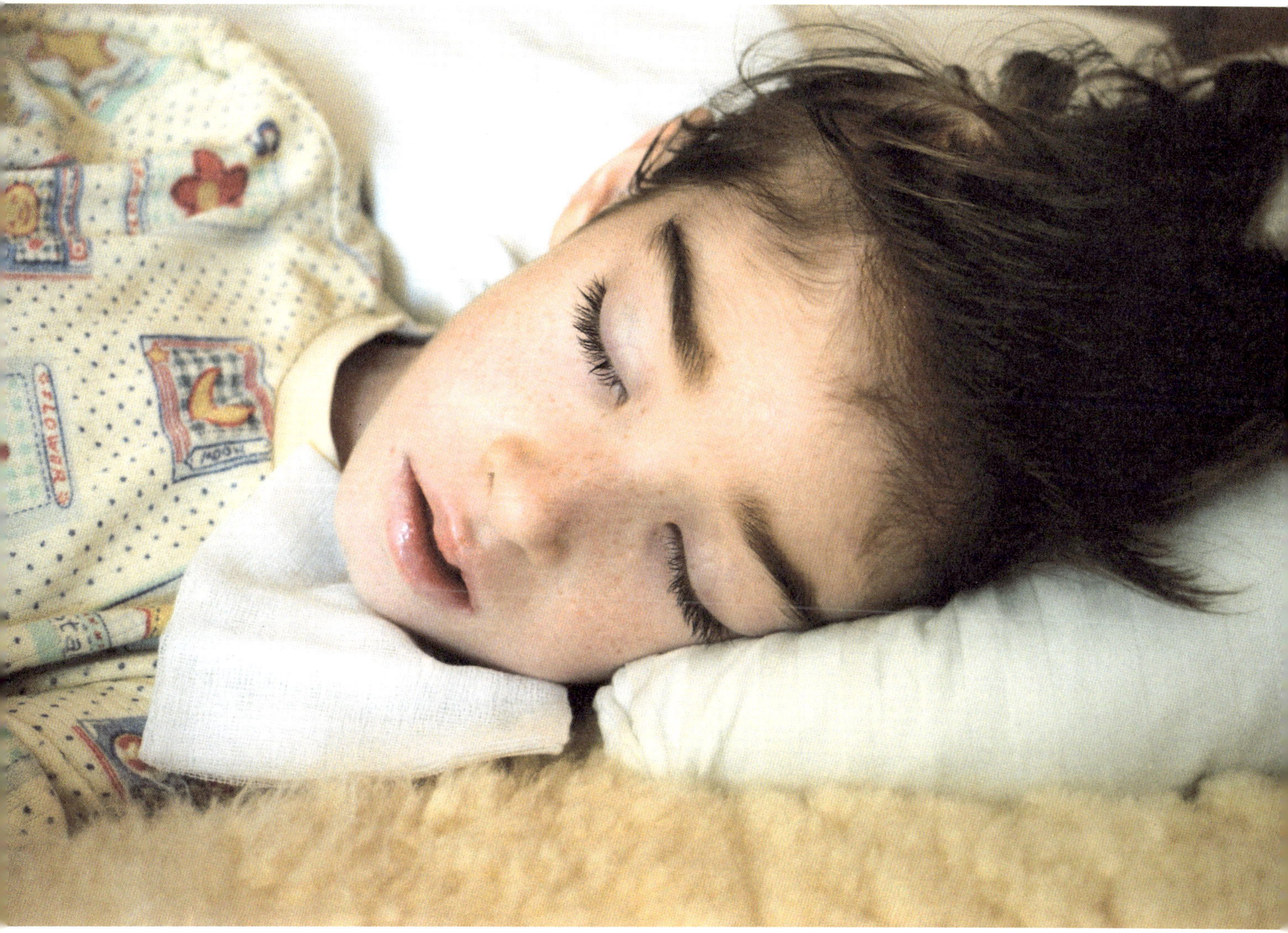

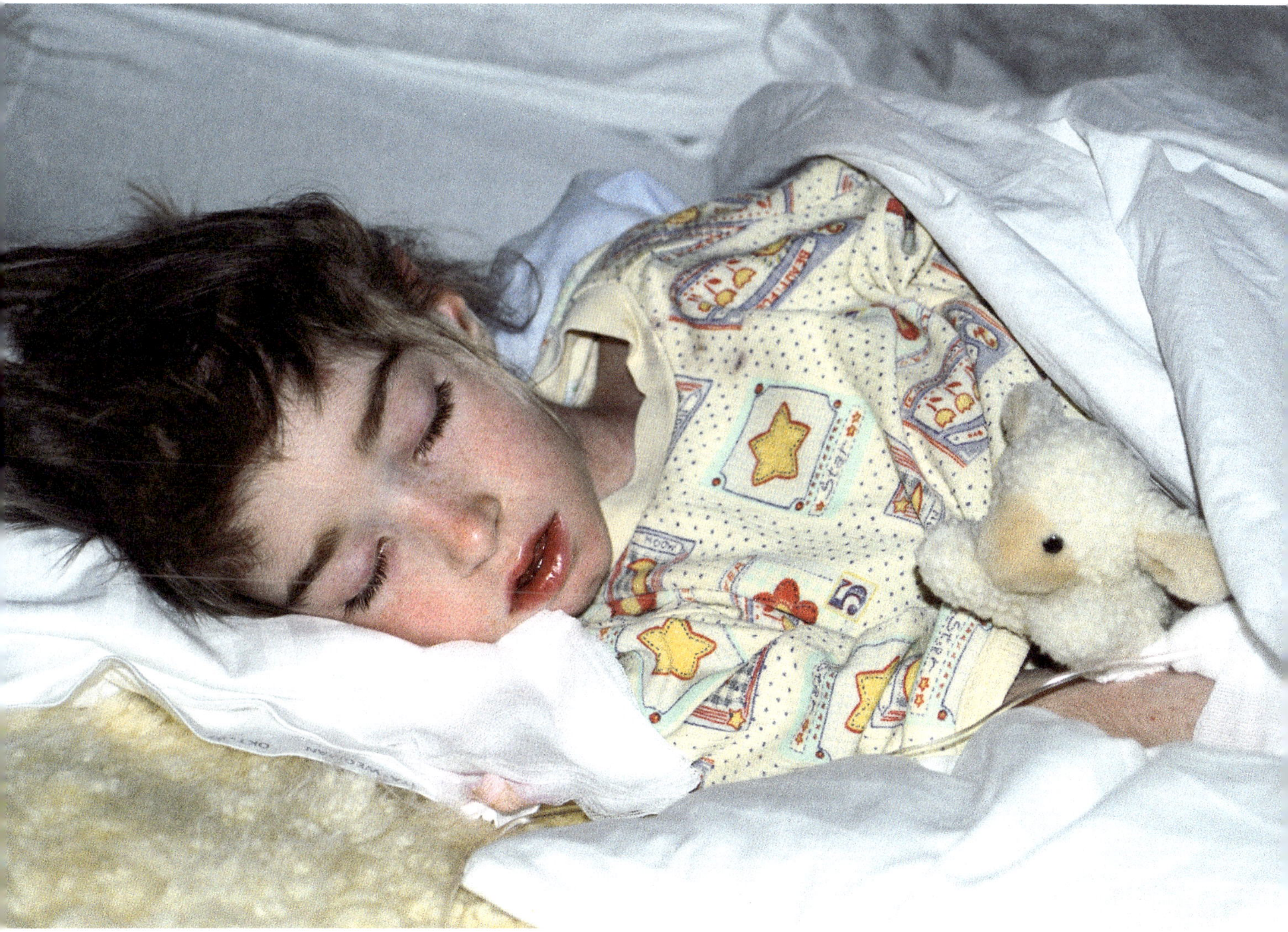

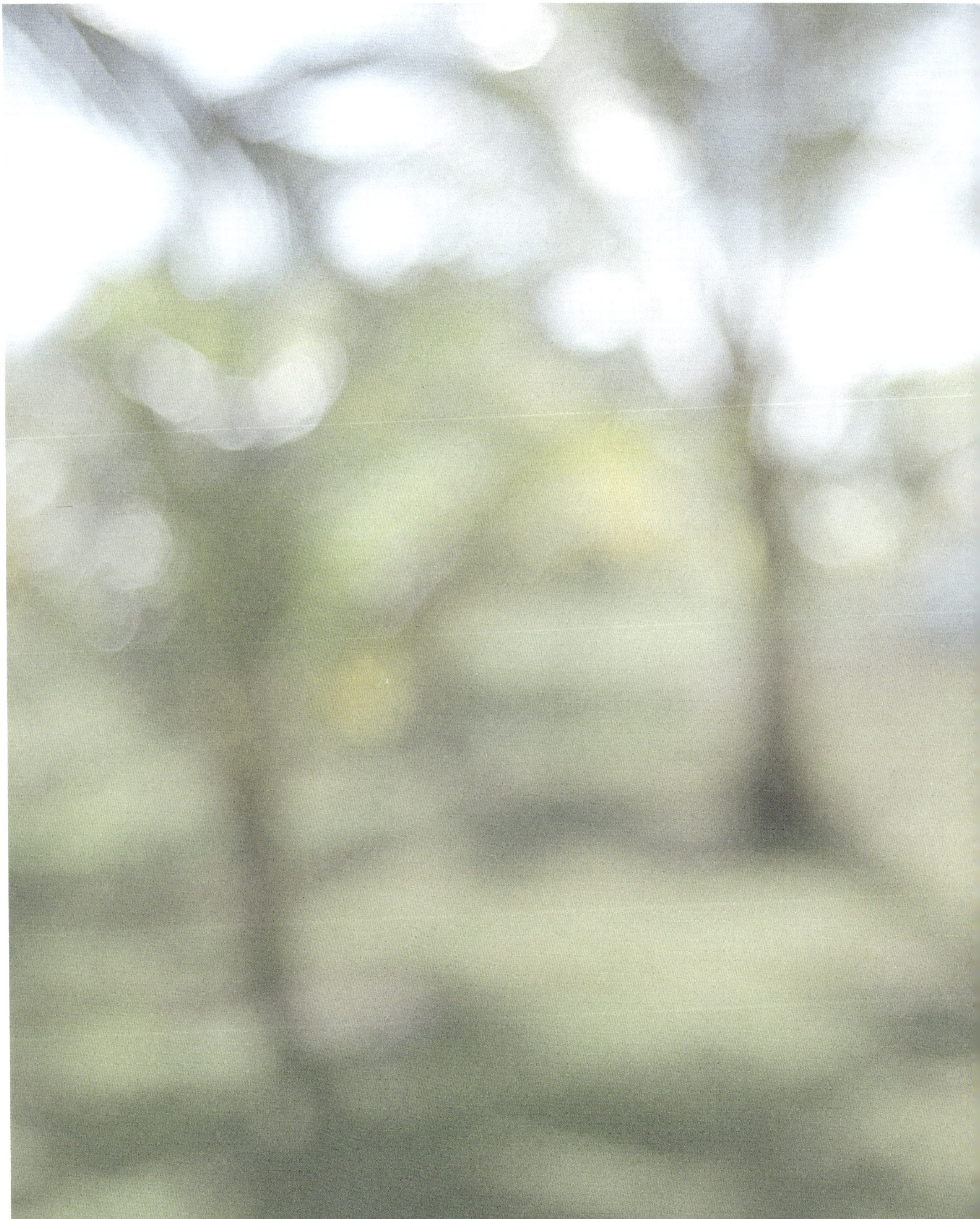

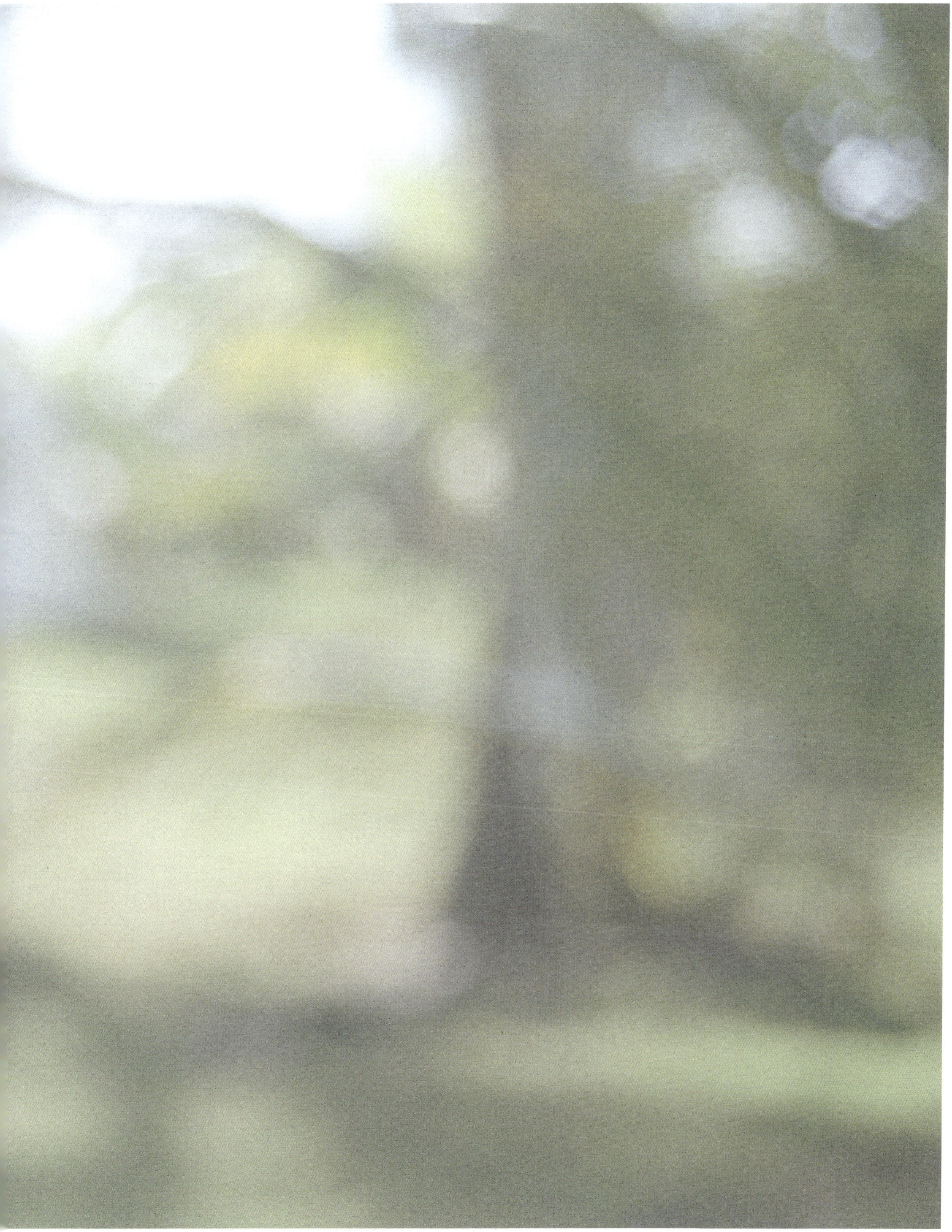

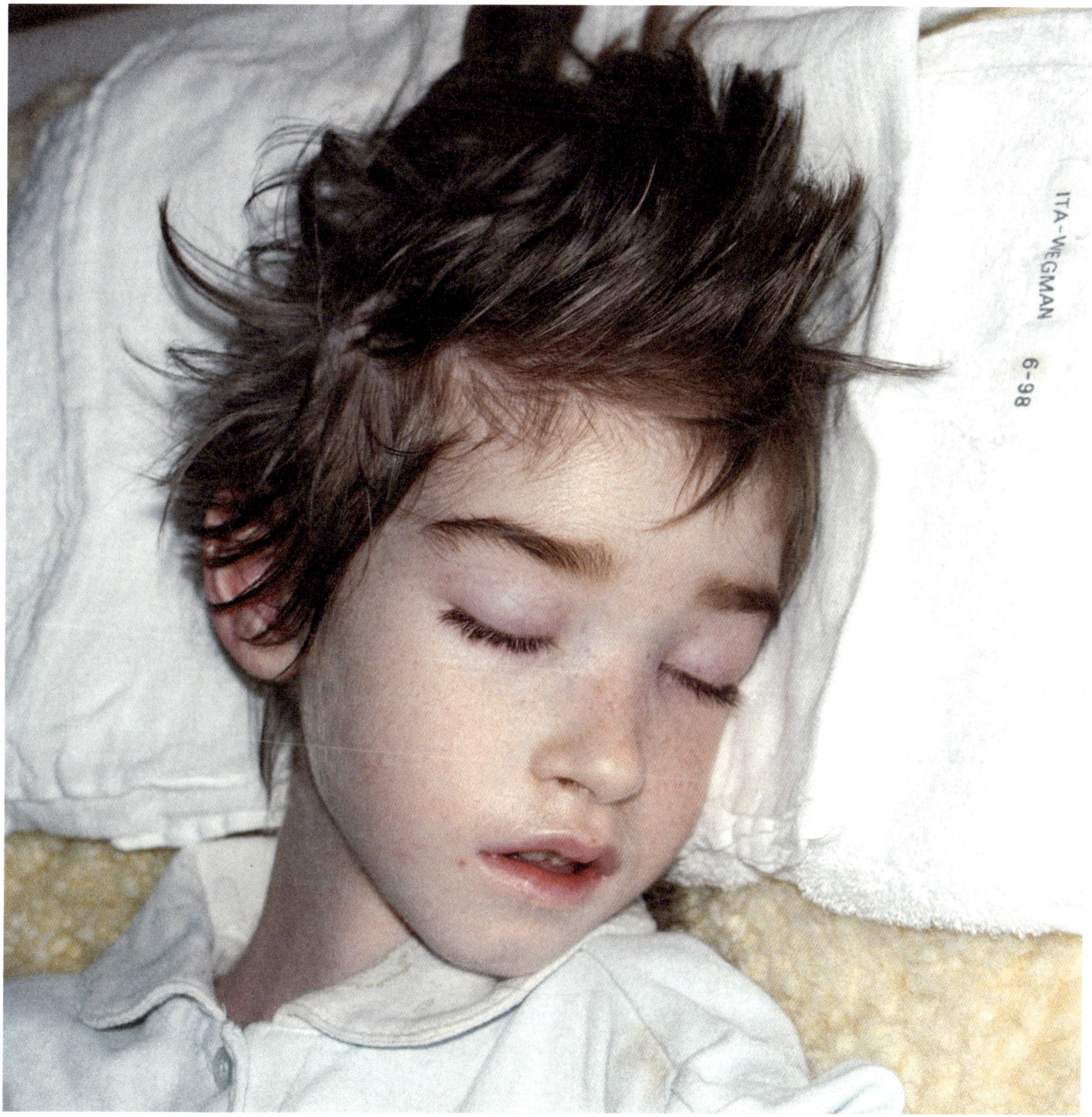
ITA-WEGMAN 6-98

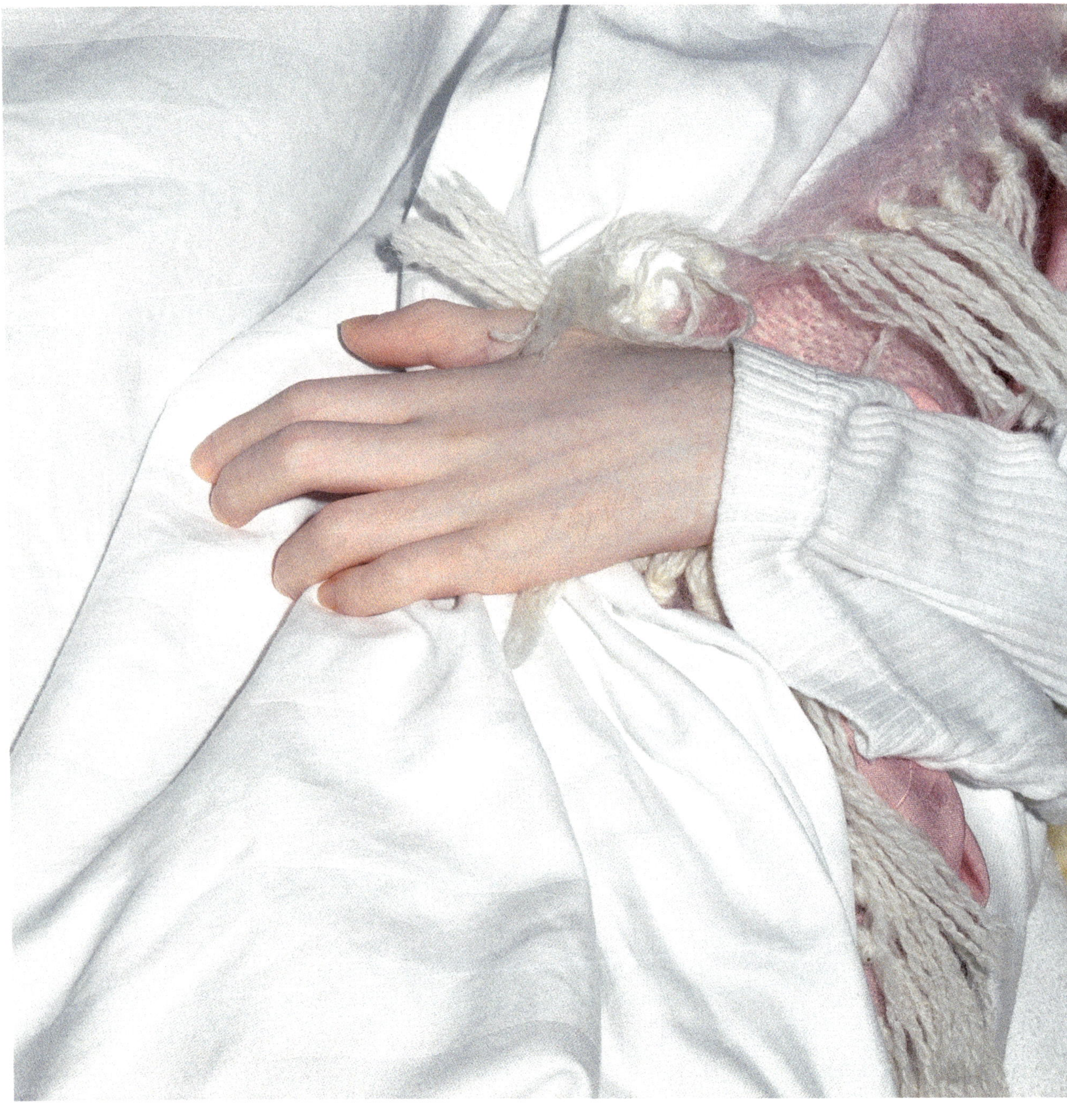

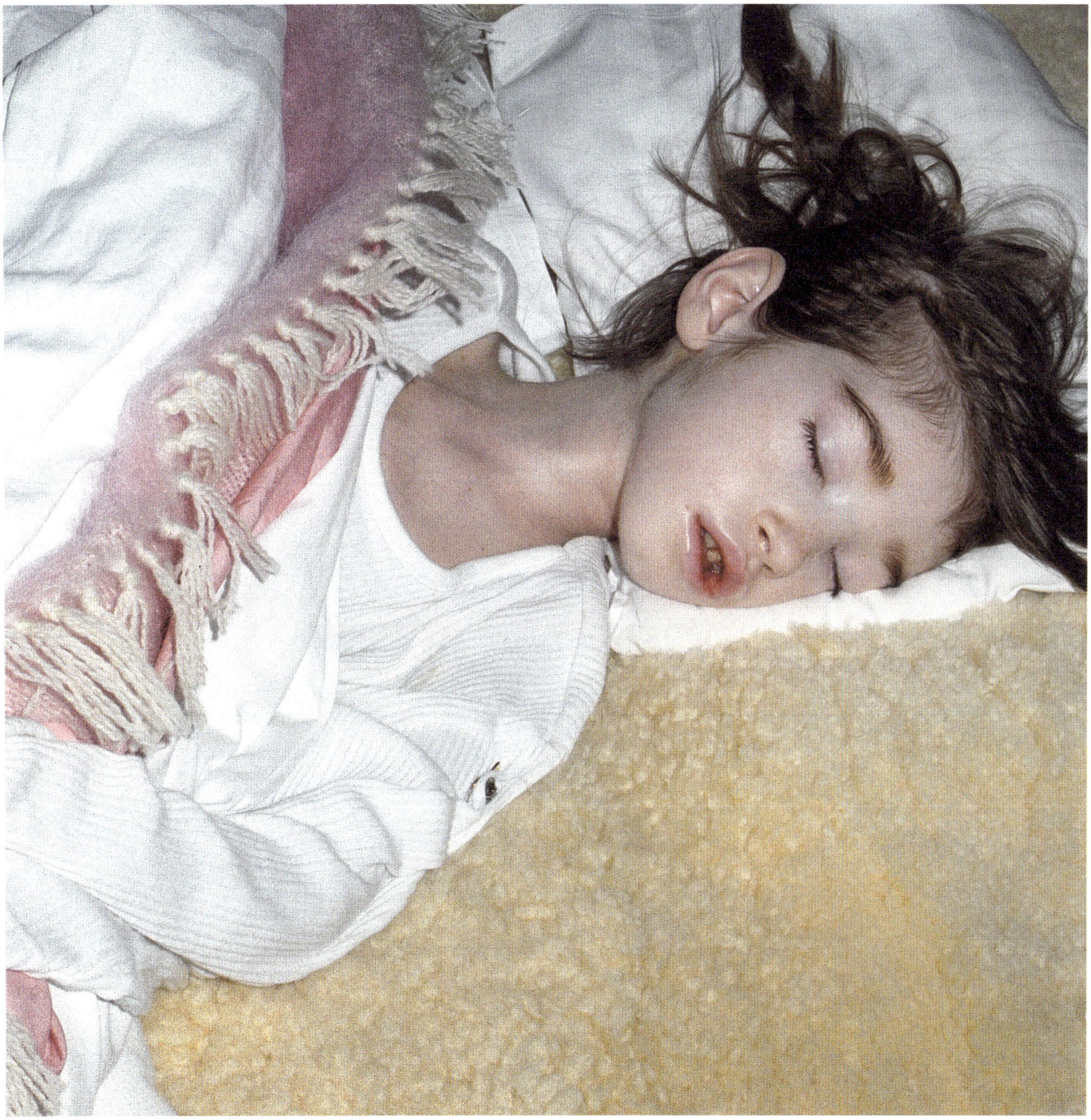

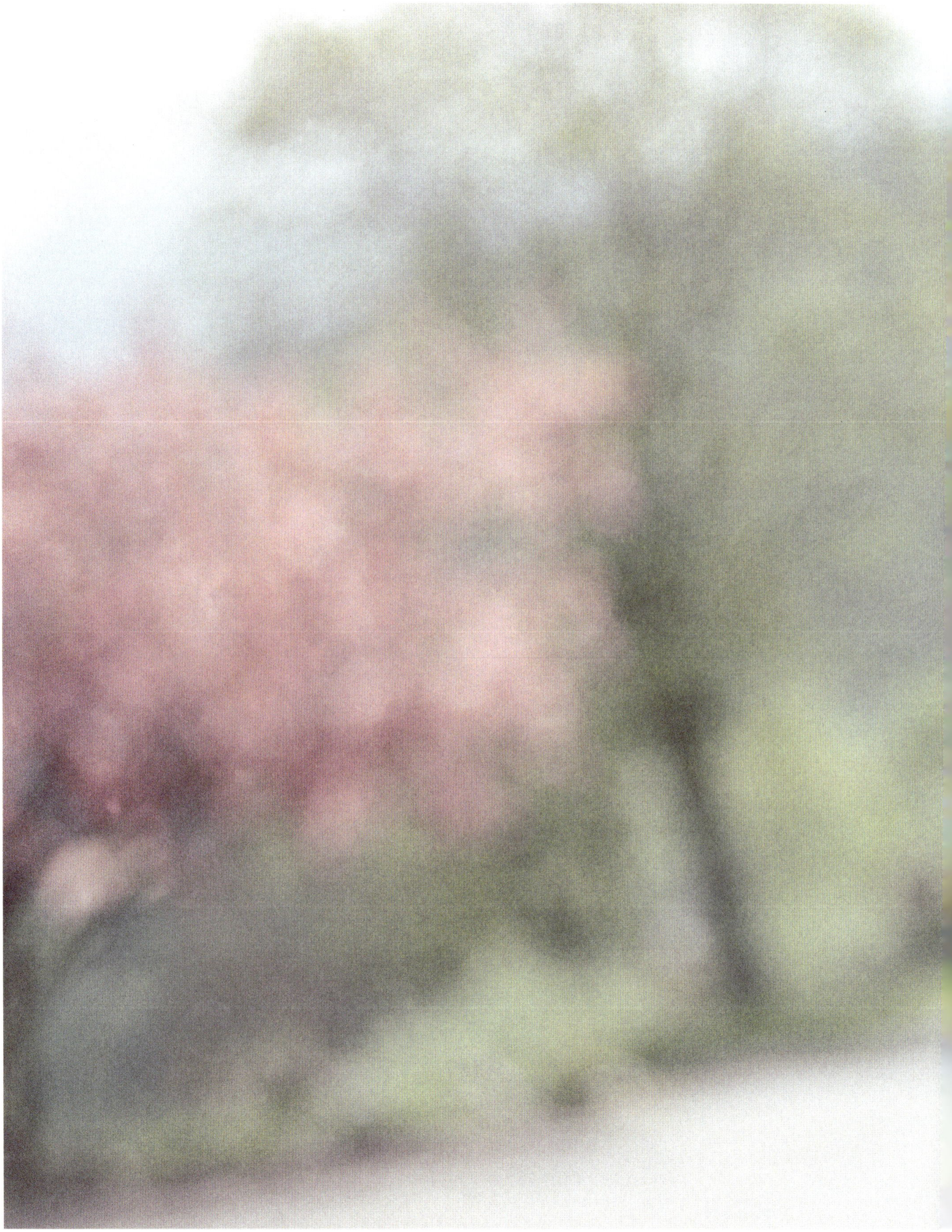

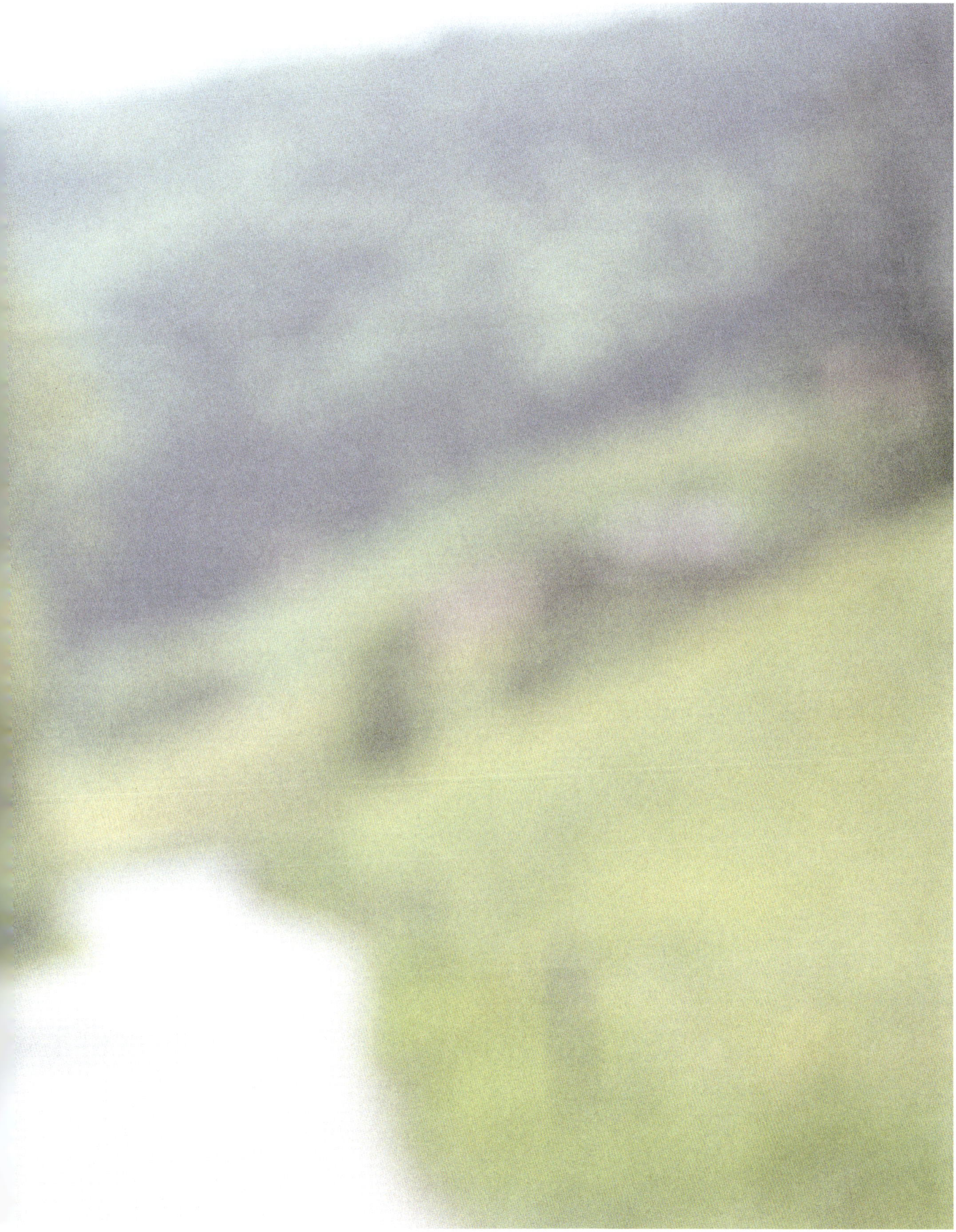

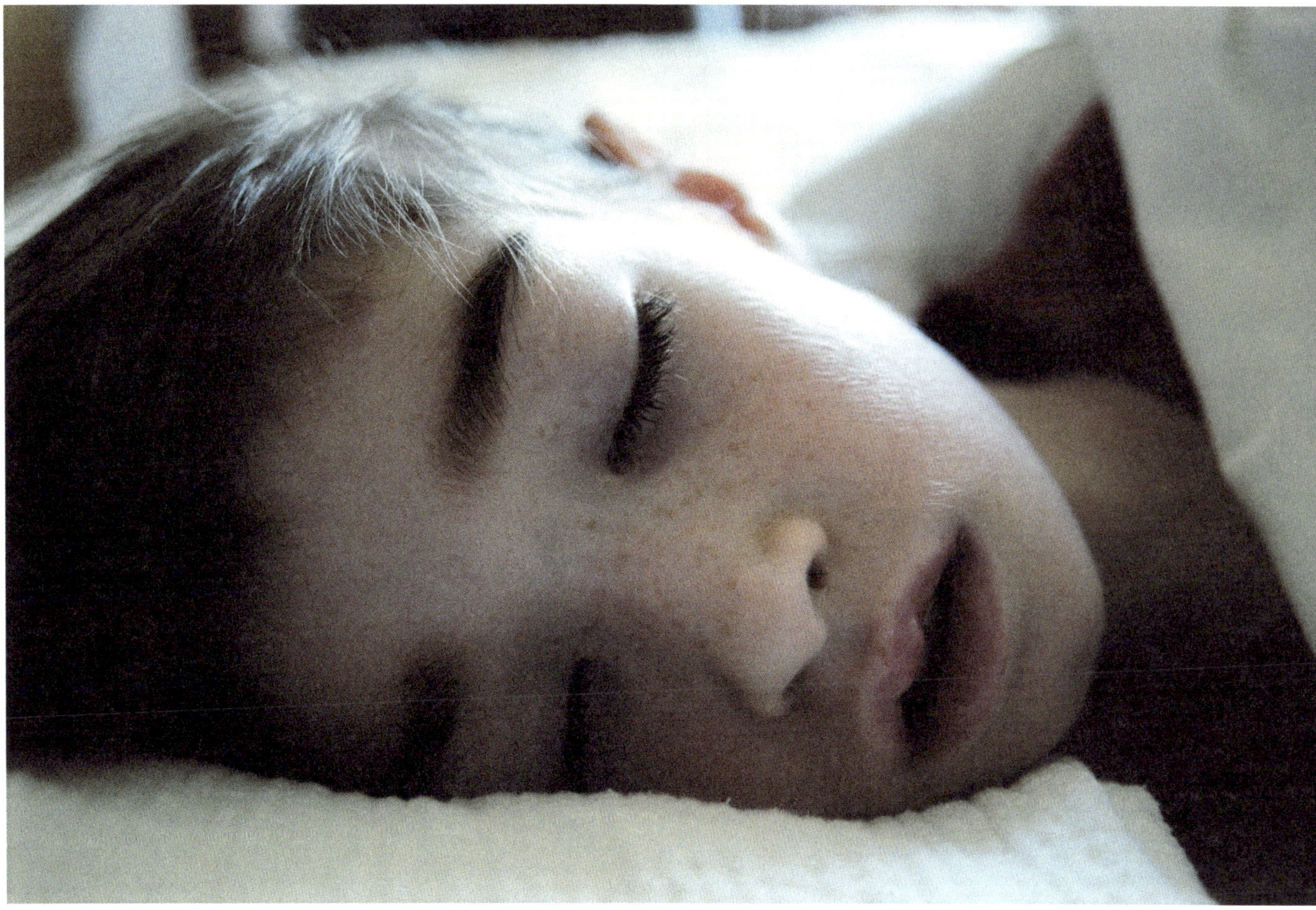

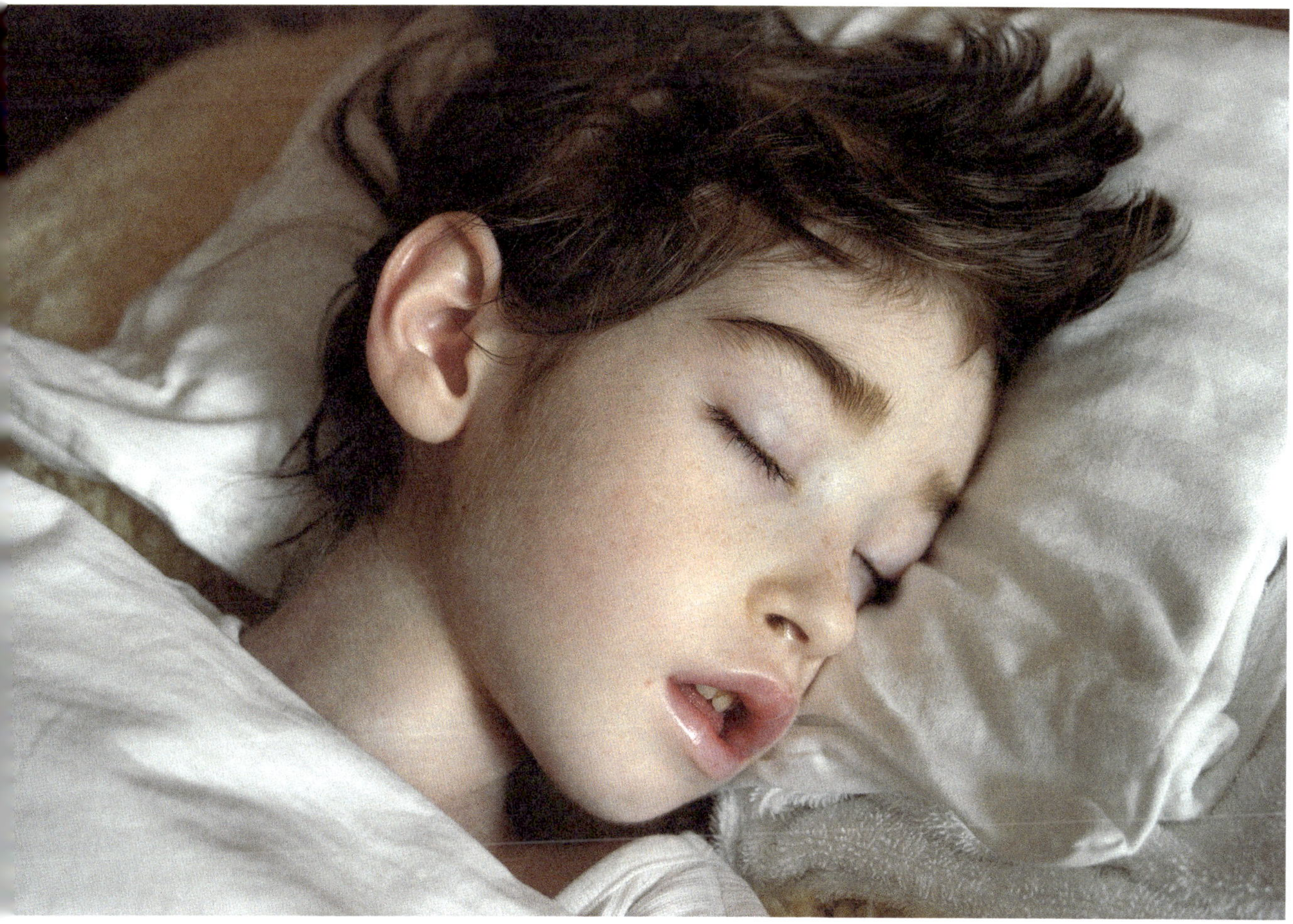

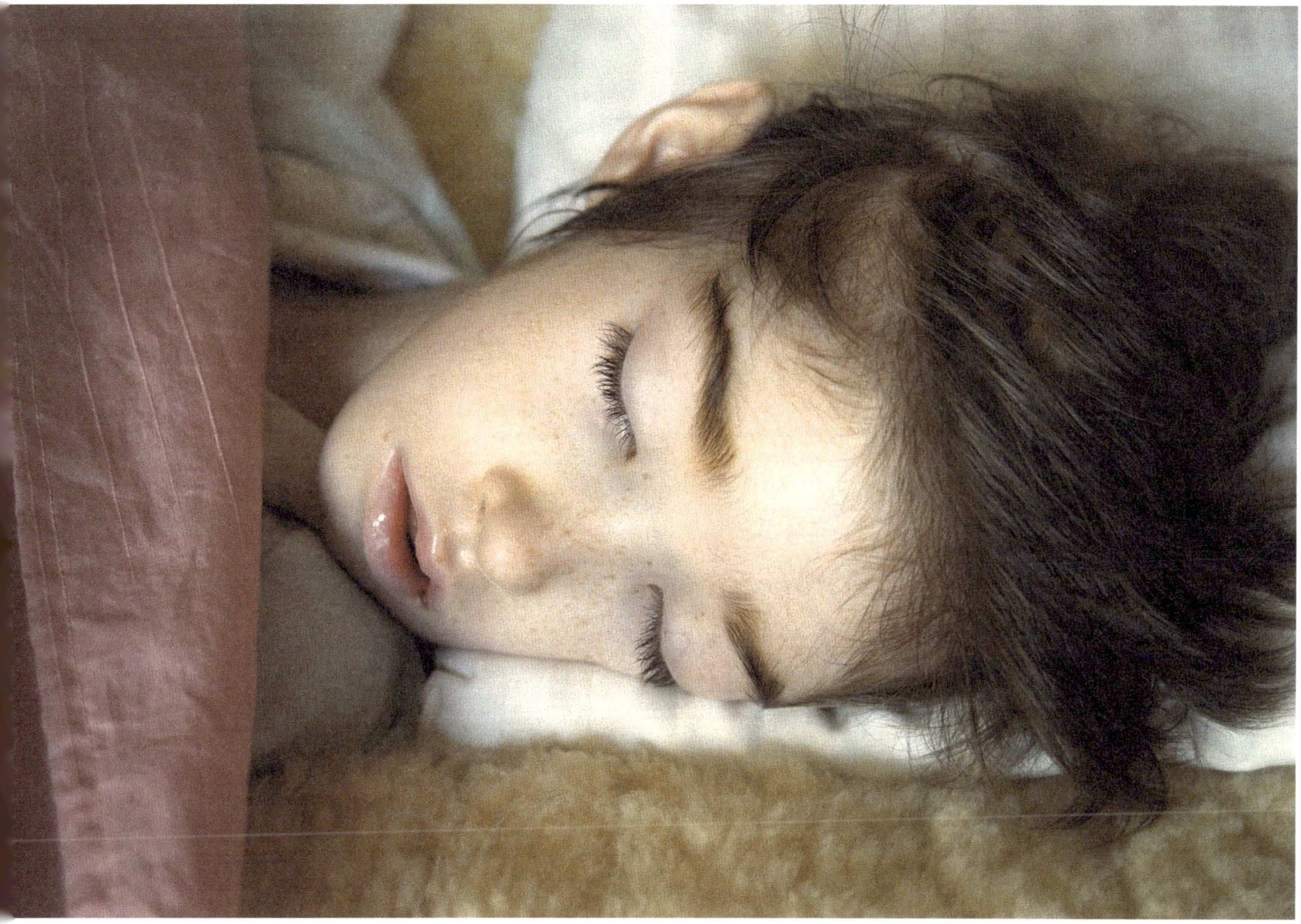

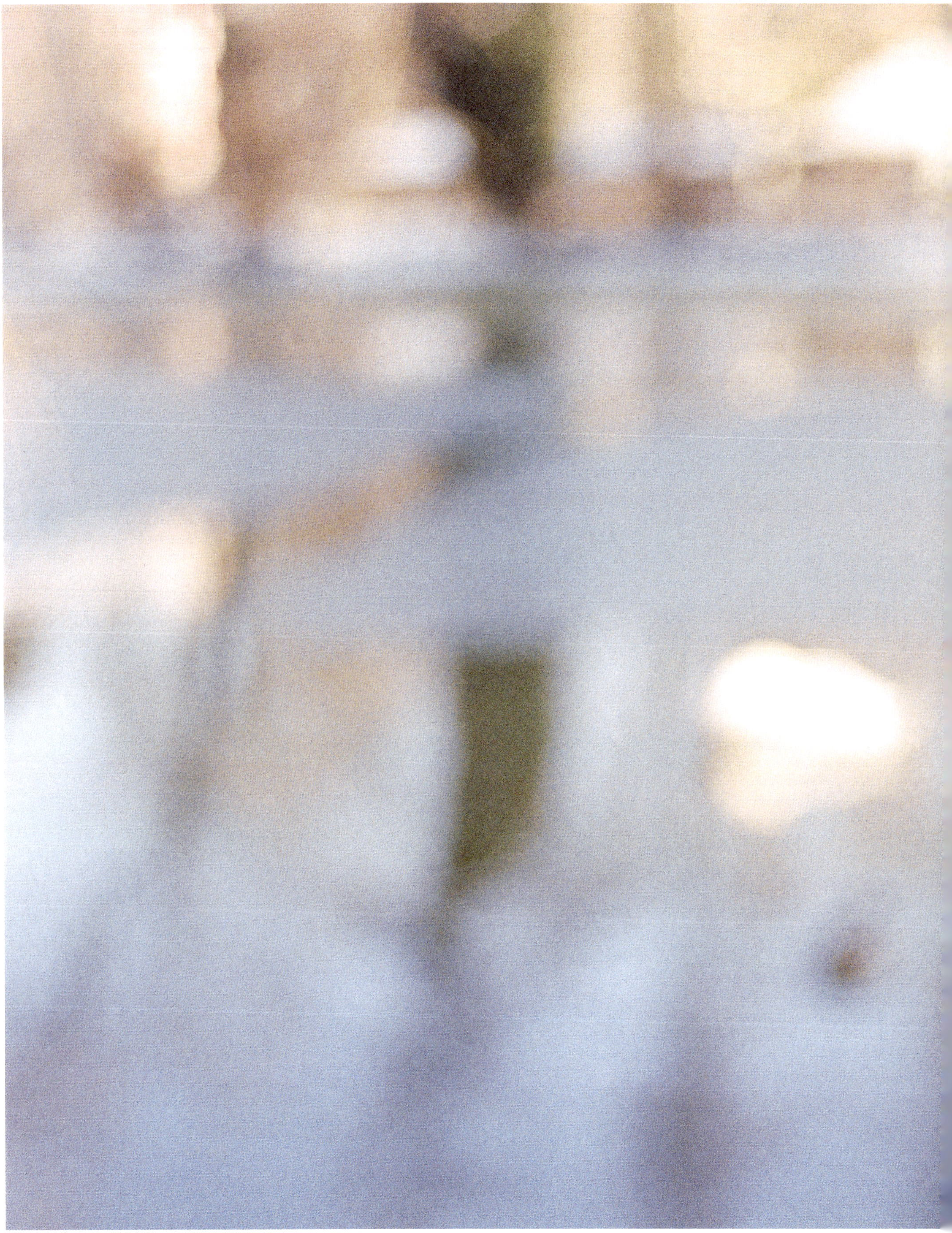

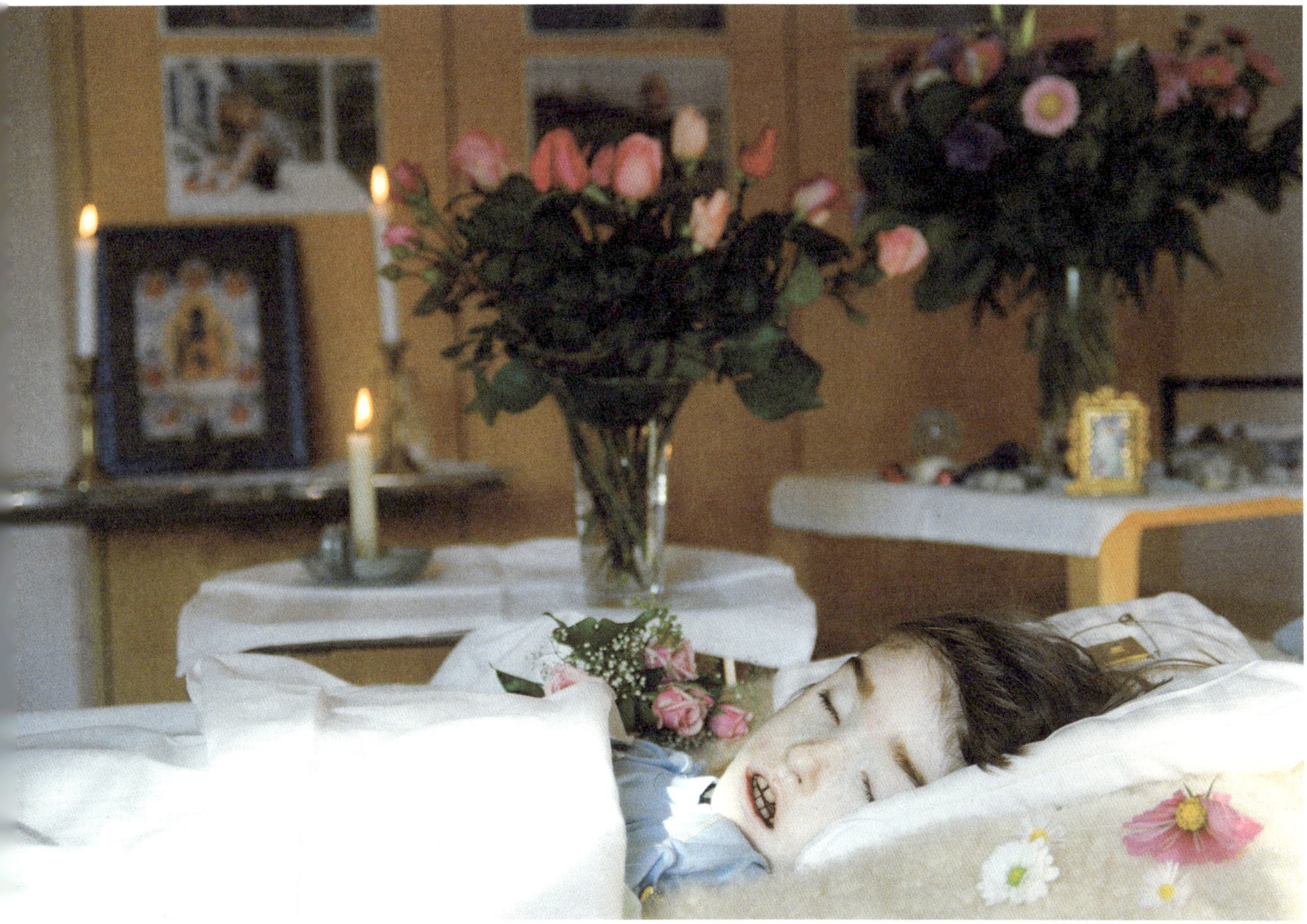

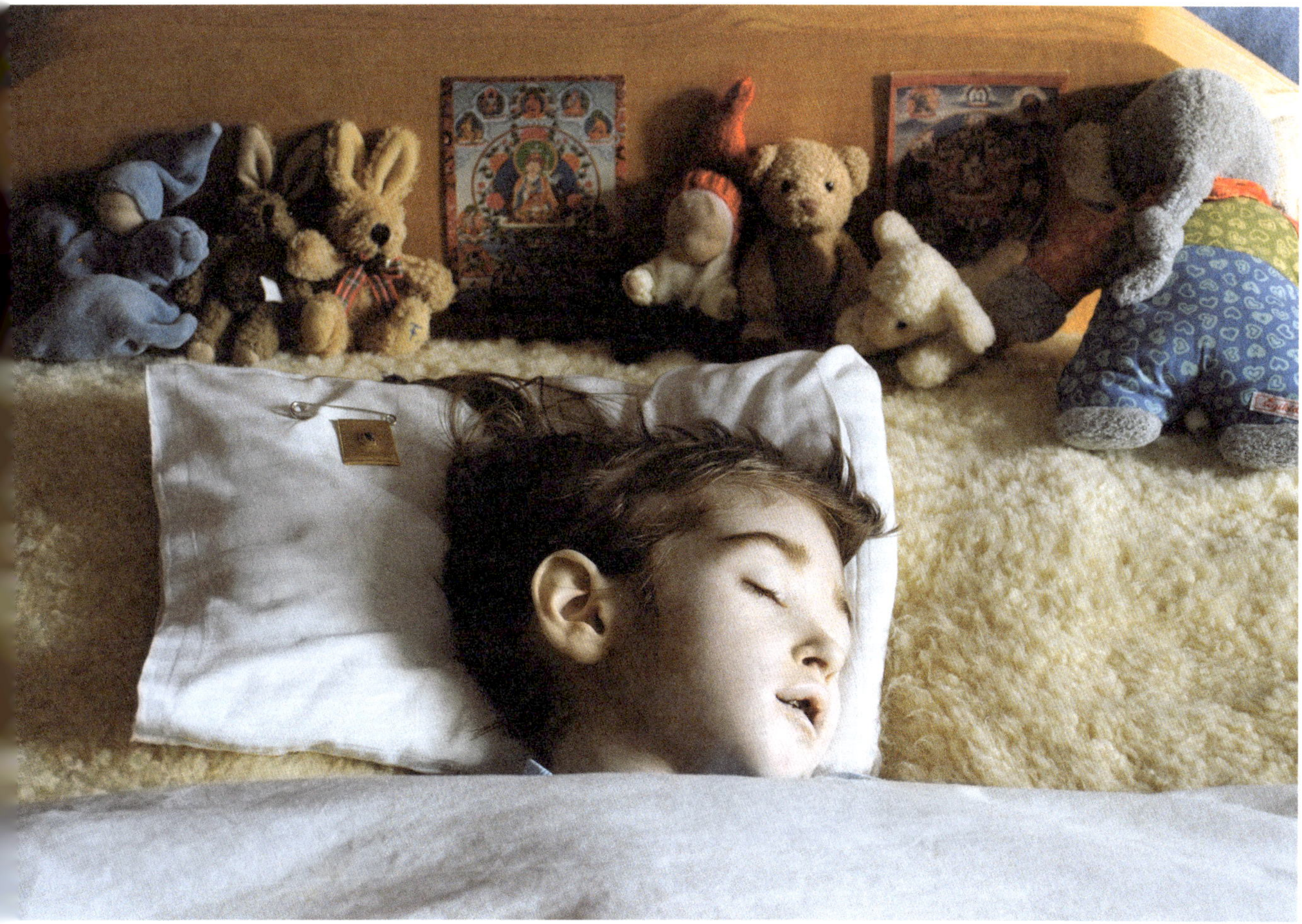

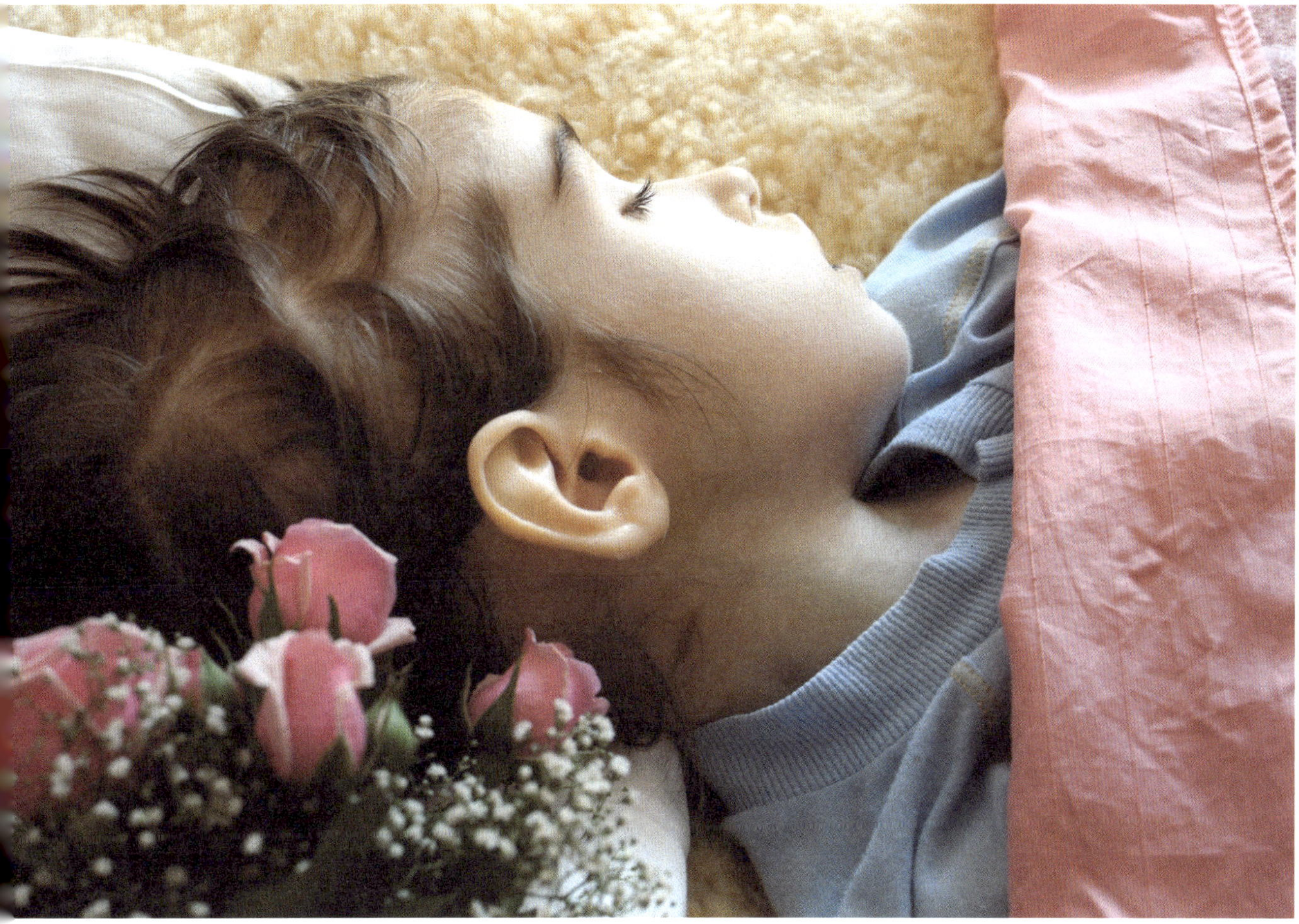

Thomas Macho

CHIARAS ABSCHIED ODER: VOM STERBEN DER KINDER

Anaximanders Satz

Die Nachricht vom Tod eines Kindes ist bestürzend. Sie erzeugt geradezu reflexartig die Frage nach fehlendem Sinn, den Vorwurf der Ungerechtigkeit, die Empfindung, dass eine Regel gebrochen wurde: die zeitliche Ordnung der Genealogie. Kinder sollten ihre Eltern bestatten, nicht umgekehrt. Die Statistik der Lebenserwartung wird heute zunehmend mit dem Natürlichen identifiziert, als würden die Gesetze der Sterblichkeit erst für ein bestimmtes Alter gelten. In solcher Perspektive bleibt der Tod stets ungerecht, «ein Beilhieb für die allermeisten, auch wenn sie alt sind»,[1] wie Ernst Bloch, wenige Wochen nach seinem 84. Geburtstag – und am Todestag Adornos – im Gespräch mit Siegfried Unseld formulierte. Oder ist das Leben selbst ungerecht, weil es immer ein Überleben ungezählter Toter miteinschliesst? Zu den ältesten Texten der europäischen Philosophie gehört ein Fragment, das dem Naturphilosophen Anaximander zugeschrieben wird, einem mutmasslichen Schüler des Thales, der um 610 bis 547 a. C. in Milet gelebt haben soll; tradiert wurde das Fragment zuletzt in den Schriften des Neuplatonikers Simplikios (6. Jahrhundert). Der dunkle Spruch des Anaximander wurde vielfach übersetzt, etwa von Friedrich Nietzsche oder Martin Heidegger; er lautete: «Woher die Dinge ihre Entstehung haben, dahin müssen sie auch zu Grunde gehen, nach der Notwendigkeit; denn sie müssen Busse zahlen und für ihre Ungerechtigkeiten gerichtet werden, gemäss der Ordnung der Zeit.»[2]

Es fällt nicht leicht, dieses Fragment angemessen zu deuten. Offenbar behauptet es eine Symmetrie von Entstehen und Vergehen, die entfernt an die indische Karma-Lehre erinnert oder an die christliche Theologie der Erbsünde; es spricht von zeitlicher Ordnung, Ungerechtigkeit und Strafe. Der Tod wird aus der Geburt abgeleitet, doch nicht im Sinne Schopenhauers, der die Frage aufwarf, warum uns die Zeit des Nichtseins vor der Geburt weniger ängstigt als die Zeit des Nichtseins nach dem Tod.[3] Im Zentrum scheint ein Unrecht zu stehen, das im Tod gebüsst wird – eine Schuld, die beglichen wird. Wer aber sind die Gläubiger? Die Ahnen und Vorfahren? Eine grosse Mutter? Ein Gott, der Welt und Menschen erschaffen hat? Die Natur, der «jeder von uns», wie Freud kritisch resümierte, einen Tod zu schulden glaubt?[4] Oder sind es die Dinge selbst, die ihren ursprünglichen Bruch mit dem *Apeiron*, dem Grenzenlosen, sühnen müssen? Und nach welchen Regeln? Unklarer noch als die Frage nach den Adressaten der Schuld bleibt die Frage nach den Kriterien der Genugtuung: Anaximanders Rekurs auf die zeitliche Ordnung. Welche Zeit und welche Ordnung? Aufzeichnungen des Kalenders oder der Generationen? Zyklen der Tage und Nächte, der Jahreszeiten, der Sterne und ihrer Konjunktionen? Listen der Namen, Geburten und Tode? Die Rede von zeitlicher Ordnung suggeriert, dass dem Endlichen – sei es Stern oder Mensch – eine Zeitspanne zugemessen ist, die nicht gesteigert werden kann. Und wenn diese Zeitspanne gar nicht erschöpft wird?

Das Ende kann vorzeitig eintreten. Die Sonne kann sich am Morgen verfinstern; Kinder können früh sterben. Zwar sind alle Menschen sterblich, doch was sie verbindet, trennt sie zugleich. Denn der Tod ist gewiss, sein Eintreten aber unbestimmt; nur *dass* wir sterben müssen, ist sicher, nicht *wie*, *wo* oder *wann*. «Mit der Gewissheit des Todes geht die Unbestimmtheit seines Wann zusammen», betonte Heidegger im § 52 von *Sein und Zeit*;[5] gerade die Differenz zwischen Gewissheit und Unbestimmtheit rücke den Tod als «eigenste Möglichkeit» des Daseins vor das innere Auge. Dem «Sein zum Tode» wird kein Alter garantiert; die einzig mögliche Antwort auf den Schrecken des vorzeitigen Todes behauptet die Einheit von Tod und

Geburt. Heidegger zitiert aus dem Streitgespräch zwischen dem böhmischen Ackermann und dem Tod: «Der Tod ist eine Weise zu sein, die das Dasein übernimmt, sobald es ist. ‹Sobald ein Mensch zum Leben kommt, sogleich ist er alt genug zu sterben.›»[6] Er verschweigt freilich, dass er aus der Rede des Todes zitiert: «ieder mensche ist vns ein sterben schuldig vnd ist in angeerbet zu sterben. Beweinestu aber deines weibes jugent, du tust vnrecht; als schiere ein mensche lebendig wirt, als schiere ist es alt genug zu sterben.»[7] Mit diesen Worten setzt sich der Tod selbst zum Gläubiger des Lebens ein, Geburtshelfer und Totengräber zugleich. «Rittlings über dem Grabe und eine schwere Geburt», kommentiert Wladimir in Samuel Becketts *Warten auf Godot*: «Aus der Tiefe der Grube legt der Totengräber träumerisch die Zangen an.»[8]

Mors immatura

Wladimirs Bemerkungen zielten auf ein westliches Publikum in der zweiten Hälfte des 20. Jahrhunderts; in anderen Epochen und Kulturen hätten sie vermutlich wenig Aufsehen erregt. *Mors immatura*, der vorzeitige Tod, gehörte zu den meistverbreiteten Plagen: Noch im Jahr 1870 starben in Deutschland 250 von 1000 Kindern, bevor sie das fünfte Lebensjahr erreicht hatten. Bis 1910 sank diese Zahl auf 160, 1927 erstmals unter 100, bis 1970 auf etwa 25; im Jahr 2006 traf die Kindersterblichkeit in Deutschland 3,8 von 1000 Kindern. Für vergangene Zeiten fehlen zumeist korrekte, statistisch auswertbare Daten. Geschätzt wird jedoch, dass noch im Mittelalter und in der frühen Neuzeit nur die Hälfte eines Jahrgangs das 21. Jahr überhaupt erlebte. Auch in der Antike war die Kindersterblichkeit so hoch, dass etwa Aristoteles behaupten konnte, es sei üblich und sinnvoll, den neugeborenen Kindern erst nach Ablauf einer Woche einen Namen zu geben, sobald «man schon eher damit rechnet, dass sie durchkommen».[9] Hauptursachen der Kindersterblichkeit waren Mangel- und Fehlernährung, Infektionen und Krankheiten (wie die Tuberkulose) oder schwere Komplikationen bei der Geburt: Querlagen, Steisslagen oder Gesichtslagen des Kindes. Zwar kamen diese Fälle nur bei etwa vier Prozent aller Geburten vor, doch bedeuteten sie stets eine erhebliche Bedrohung des Lebens der Mutter und des Kindes,[10] der oft nur mit aussergewöhnlichen Massnahmen – wie der berüchtigten Embryotomie, der Zerstückelung des Kindes im Mutterleib[11] – begegnet werden konnte.

Die Statistik bedarf der Konkretisierung. 24 Kinder zeugte der spanische Maler Francisco de Goya – lange bevor er seinen grauenhaften Saturn malte (1820–1823) – mit Josefa Bayeu: Ein einziger Sohn, Xavier, überlebte. In einer Ausgabe der Werke des Grafen Friedrich von Hardenberg, besser bekannt unter seinem Dichternamen Novalis, findet sich ein Stammbaum, eine schlichte Zusammenstellung der Namen und Daten, die vor mehr als zweihundert Jahren eine Familie gebildet haben;[12] daraus geht hervor: Novalis selbst ist am 25. März 1801 gestorben, im 29. Lebensjahr. Von seinen zehn Geschwistern wurden nur zwei Brüder älter als dreissig Jahre – Carl und Georg Anton, die mit 37 und 44 Jahren auch nicht gerade ein biblisches Alter erreichten. Im Jahr 1818 – dem Todesjahr der Mutter – war nicht nur sein Vater schon seit vier Jahren tot, sondern nur noch ein einziger Sohn von elf Kindern am Leben. Nebenbei vermerkt: Die Verlobte des Dichters, Sophie von Kühn, starb zwei Tage nach ihrem 15. Geburtstag. Der Dichter Friedrich Rückert verlor seine beiden jüngsten Kinder, Luise und Ernst, innerhalb von wenigen Wochen – am 31. Dezember 1833 und am 16. Januar 1834 – durch Scharlach; danach schrieb er die von Gustav Mahler 1901 und 1904 vertonten *Kindertotenlieder*. Giuseppe Verdis gesamte Familie – Tochter und Sohn, jeweils im Alter von 16 Monaten, dann die Ehefrau – starb innerhalb von zwei Jahren, zwischen 1838 und 1840. Der tschechische Komponist Antonin Dvořák schliesslich begann in Trauer um den Tod seiner Tochter Josefa (sie starb am 19. Dezember 1875, zwei Tage nach der Geburt) die Arbeit an seinem grossen Oratorium *Stabat Mater*; noch vor Vollendung dieses Werks am 13. November 1877 waren auch die elfmonatige Tochter Ruzena und der dreijährige Sohn Otakar (im August 1877) gestorben.

Es fällt schwer, sich in ein Bewusstsein einzufühlen, das eine solche Sequenz von Abschieden erlitten und überlebt hat. Daher ist auch nicht verwunderlich, dass manche Historiker die Meinung vertreten haben, der Wert eines Kinderlebens sei in älteren Kulturen nicht hoch eingeschätzt worden;[13] erst die jüngste Moderne habe allmählich gelernt, um gestorbene Kinder zu trauern. Solche Vermutungen sind schwer widerlegbar;[14] doch können sie an einzelnen Beispielen ein wenig relativiert werden. So schrieb Plutarch – nach dem Tod der zweijährigen Tochter – einen Trostbrief an seine Gattin Timoxena, in dem er betonte, er sei nicht «aus Eichen und Steinen gemacht», sondern kenne ihren Schmerz: «Ich weiss, dass diese Tochter, deren Geburt nach vier Söhnen deinen sehnlichsten Wunsch erfüllte und mich veranlasste, ihr deinen Namen zu geben, dir ganz besonders lieb war. Was deine zärtliche Liebe zu dem Kinde noch besonders steigerte, ist die reine, unschuldige, niemals durch Ärger und Tadel getrübte Freude, die es uns machte.»[15] Plutarch glaubte an die Unsterblichkeit der Seele. Im Schreiben an seine Frau betonte er, dass die Gesetze es nicht gestatten, «Tote von solchem Alter zu betrauern»;[16] zugleich versicherte er ihr: «Unsere Tochter aber, welche sich an einem Ort befindet, wo es keinen Schmerz mehr gibt, braucht uns keine Sorge zu machen».[17] Rund 1500 Jahre später schickte Michel de Montaigne eine Übersetzung dieses Trostbriefs an seine eigene Frau, als er die Nachricht vom Tod der ältesten Tochter erhielt.

Kindertotenbilder

Nach christlicher Tradition wurde die Taufe eines Kindes, seine Integration in die Kirche, für wichtiger gehalten als seine Gesundheit oder ein langes Leben. Es ging ja um das himmlische Heil und den künftigen Aufenthalt seiner unsterblichen Seele. Starb das Kind bald nach der Geburt – was häufig genug passierte –, war es daher möglich, den Weg in die nächste Kirche anzutreten und ein Gnadenbild der Gottesmutter oder eines Heiligen zu bitten, das Kind zu «zeichnen»; an sichtbaren Zeichen (wie geröteten Wangen, Atemgeräuschen oder kleinen Zuckungen) sollte jener kurze Moment erkannt werden, für den es ins Leben zurückgerufen wurde, um rasch getauft werden zu können. Die ehemalige Marienkapelle von Oberbüren im Kanton Bern war im Spätmittelalter ein bekanntes Zentrum der Schweiz, an dem gestorbene Kinder auf diese Weise wieder «zum Leben erweckt» werden konnten. Bischof Otto von Sonnenberg († 1491) beschrieb diese Praxis mit folgenden Worten: Die «Frauen erwärmten die todten Kinder zwischen glühenden Kohlen und ringsum hingestellten brennenden Kerzen und Lichtern. Dem warm gewordenen todten Kinde oder der Frühgeburt wird eine ganz leichte Feder über die Lippen gelegt und wenn die Feder zufällig durch die Luft oder die Wärme der Kohlen von den Lippen weg bewegt wird, so erklären die Weiber, die Kinder und Frühgeburten atmeten und lebten und sofort lassen sie dieselben taufen unter Glockengeläute und Lobgesängen. Die Körper der angeblich lebendig gewordenen und sofort wieder verstorbenen Kinder lassen sie dann kirchlich beerdigen.»[18] Die Marienkapelle wurde in den Zeiten der Reformation abgerissen und erst vor wenigen Jahren archäologisch untersucht; dabei wurde die «Chilchmatt» freigelegt, eine Bestattungsfläche von mehr als 3500 Quadratmetern, die schon seit der späten Bronzezeit genutzt wurde. An mehreren Stellen entdeckten die Archäologen Begräbnisflächen für mehr als 250 nach der Geburt verstorbene Kinder, die offenbar im Moment ihrer kurzen «Wiedererweckung» getauft wurden, wie aus der Körperhaltung der kleinen Skelette mit ihren gekreuzten Armen und der Ausrichtung der Grablage nach Jerusalem geschlossen werden darf.

Das «Kinderzeichnen» bildete eine religiöse Praxis, die allmählich in Vergessenheit geriet; erst solches Vergessen ermöglichte den Vorwurf, mittelalterliche Eltern hätten ihre toten Kinder nicht betrauert. Im anbrechenden Zeitalter der Säkularisierung und Religionskritik wurde der spirituelle Trost, der oft nicht mehr überzeugend gewährt werden konnte, durch künstlerische Ausdrucksformen der Trauer ersetzt. Die toten Kinder wurden nun tatsächlich gezeichnet oder gemalt: Charles Willson

Peale malte etwa seine Frau und die verstorbene Tochter Margaret als *Rachel Weeping* (1772–1776);[19] der Wiener Maler Friedrich von Amerling porträtierte nicht nur 1843 seine Frau Antonie am Sterbebett, sondern sieben Jahre später auch den gemeinsamen Sohn Fritz.[20] Nach Erfindung der Fotografie etablierten sich Ateliers in den nordamerikanischen und europäischen Metropolen, die – häufig in Kooperation mit der Friedhofsverwaltung und den jeweiligen Bestattungsinstituten – die letzten Bilder der Toten produzierten: als Andenken und Erinnerungszeichen, später auch als Elemente von Grabsteinen.[21] Um 1850 erbot sich Félix Nadar, Pionier der Daguerreotypie, Totenfotos in seinem Pariser Atelier anzufertigen. In München warb Adolph Scheuerer 1858 mit dem Versprechen «grösster Ähnlichkeit» und einem «freundlichen Anblick» seiner Leichenporträts um neue Aufträge; auf dem Münchener Südfriedhof wurden bereits 1857 mehr als dreihundert Verstorbene im offenen Sarg abgelichtet. In Wien reüssierte der Fotograf Albin Mutterer, der erstmals in Nussdorf ein glasgedecktes Atelier errichten liess, als Spezialist für das neue Genre der Totenfotografie.[22]

Jay Ruby hat in seiner Studie zu *Death and Photography in America* mehrere Typen der Totenabbildung im 19. Jahrhundert unterschieden: die «Alive, yet dead»-Bilder, die den Verstorbenen in aufrechter Haltung, oft mit retuschierten Augen, darstellen, die «Last Sleep»-Bilder, die den Toten scheinbar im Schlaf – etwa auf einer Bettbank oder in einer Wiege – zeigen, und schliesslich die Fotografien des Toten im offenen Sarg.[23] Auf zahlreichen Bildern sieht man die Angehörigen der Toten, in einigen Fällen sogar die gesamte Trauergemeinde, was jedenfalls das zynische Aperçu widerlegt, wonach die ältere Fotografie mit ihren langen Belichtungszeiten die Totenporträts bevorzugt habe, weil Leichen keine Bilder verwackeln. Die meisten Totenfotos, die Jay Ruby (oder Stanley B. Burns[24]) gesammelt haben, präsentieren übrigens verstorbene Kinder; zu Recht betonte Philippe Ariès: «Kaum ein Familienalbum bleibt ohne Photos toter Kinder. [...] Der Tod des Kindes ist der erste unerträgliche Tod. Kindergrabmäler waren vor dem 16. Jahrhundert inexistent oder aussergewöhnlich; sie bleiben auch im 17. selten und linkisch. Im 19. Jahrhundert erobern sich die Kinder dagegen die Friedhöfe. Man spürt, dass man darauf bedacht gewesen ist, sie in allen erdenklichen Haltungen darzustellen, um den starken Schmerz der Eltern und ihr leidenschaftliches Bedürfnis zum Ausdruck zu bringen, ihnen im Gedenken und in der Kunst ein Nachleben zu sichern, ihre Unschuld, ihren Charme und ihre Schönheit schwärmerisch zu übersteigern.»[25]

Chiaras Abschied

Keine Spur solcher «schwärmerischen Übersteigerung» findet sich in den Fotos, die Elisabeth Zahnd Legnazzi von ihrer Tochter Chiara – während eines langsamen Sterbens – gemacht hat. Die Sequenz der Bilder bezeugt den Abschied des Kindes, einen allmählichen Rückzug von der Welt: Sichtbar wird der Blick, der kein Gegenüber mehr findet. In seiner *Anthropologie in pragmatischer Hinsicht* (1798) hatte Immanuel Kant den Tod als Endpunkt einer Serie von Sinnesverlusten bestimmt, die den Rausch mit dem Schlaf und die Ohnmacht mit dem Scheintod assoziiert: als «Vorspiel» des Todes; er hat aber auch den unüberwindlichen Abstand betont, der noch die extremste Bewusstlosigkeit vom tatsächlichen Eintritt des Todes trennt. «Das Sterben kann kein Mensch an sich selbst erfahren (denn eine Erfahrung zu machen, dazu gehört Leben), sondern nur an andern wahrnehmen.»[26] Ich kann sehen, dass ich nicht mehr gesehen werde; darin liegt die tiefe Kränkung, die den Überlebenden zugefügt wird. In seiner Totenrede auf Peter Noll hat Max Frisch am 18. Oktober 1982 bemerkt: «Wir sind zur Trauer versammelt. Einen Verstorbenen öffentlich zu loben und öffentlich zu versichern, dass man ihn vermissen werde, ist der übliche Ausdruck unserer redlichen Trauer in Ahnungslosigkeit, was Tod ist. Kein Antlitz in einem Sarg hat mir je gezeigt, dass der Eben-Verstorbene uns vermisst. Das Gegenteil davon ist überdeutlich. [...] Der Verstorbene überlässt mich der Erinnerung an meine Erlebnisse mit ihm ...»[27]

Im Übergang zwischen Schlafen und Wachen scheint Chiara nicht zu sehen, dass sie gesehen und fotografiert wird; umgekehrt scheint sie ihrerseits zu sehen, was die Fotografin gar nicht sehen kann. Auf diese Weise entzieht sich das Gesicht des Kindes jeder Verführung zur Pose; es avanciert zum «Nicht-Porträt» (nach einem Ausdruck von Charlotte Klonk[28]). Ein «Nicht-Porträt» bricht den Kontrakt der Repräsentation: das Versprechen einer Vergegenwärtigung, die als *geteilte* Zeit zwischen dem Betrachter und dem Betrachteten erfahren wird. Was aber zeigt ein Gesicht, das nicht zu sehen scheint, dass es gesehen wird? Es demonstriert nicht die eigene Abwesenheit, sondern die Abwesenheit der Anderen. Umso dringlicher muss es begleitet werden: seltener von Vater oder Mutter, manchmal von Blumen oder einem Stofftier. Am Ende werden die Blumen und die Galerie der Kuscheltiere – kaum weniger anrührend als eine menschliche Trauergemeinde – über das tote Mädchen wachen. Warum erschüttert gerade die Präsenz der Dinge? Warum beschwor schon Plutarch das «liebreiche Wesen» seiner verstorbenen Tochter, indem er sich daran erinnerte, wie das Kind «seine Amme bat, nicht nur andern Kindern, sondern selbst Gerätschaften und Spielsachen, an denen es eine Freude hatte, die Brust zu reichen, ganz so, wie wenn es sie aus Menschenliebe an seinen eigenen Tisch zur Teilnahme an seinen Genüssen einladen und mit denen, welche ihr Freude machten, sein Süssestes teilen wollte»?[29] Dinge sind Medien der Verwandlung, Brücken zwischen Person und materieller Welt; häufig sind es gerade Spielsachen, die als letzte Gaben die Kinder in den Sarg begleiten oder ihre Grabstellen schmücken.[30]

Zwischen den «Nicht-Porträts» des Mädchens Chiara (wörtlich: die Glänzende, die Helle – was in ihrem zweiten Vornamen: *Lucia*, die Leuchtende, das Licht, noch ergänzt wird) erscheinen mehrfach unscharfe Fotos, deren Gegenstände – farbige Flächen, Lichtpunkte, Innen- und Aussenräume – nicht deutlich erkannt werden können. Die grossflächigen Bilder, die nichts abbilden, referieren auf die nachlassende Sehkraft des Kindes; sie können aber auch auf jene *Reise ins Licht* bezogen werden, die der Untertitel des Buchs ankündigt. Dieser Untertitel verweist einerseits auf jene häufig zitierten Nahtodberichte, die eine Art von Geburtserfahrung darzustellen scheinen: die Fahrt durch einen Tunnel, an dessen Ende ein strahlendes Licht wahrgenommen wird, andererseits aber auf das Wesen der Fotografie selbst. Seit ihrer Erfindung ist die Kunst der Aufzeichnung von Lichtbildern mit dem Tod assoziiert worden. In solchem Sinne schrieb etwa Roland Barthes vom Schrecken des Todes, «dass es nichts zu sagen gibt über den Tod des Menschen, den ich am meisten liebe, nichts über sein Photo, das ich betrachte, ohne es je ausloten, umwandeln zu können.»[31] Denn der Tod ist so kontingent wie jeder Augenblick, dem das Foto eine dauerhafte Gestalt verleiht. «Fotografieren heisst die Sterblichkeit inventarisieren», bemerkte Susan Sontag. «Fotografien konstatieren die Unschuld, die Verletzlichkeit, die Ahnungslosigkeit von Menschen, die ihrer eigenen Vernichtung entgegengehen, und gerade die Verknüpfung zwischen Fotografie und Tod verleiht allen Aufnahmen von Menschen etwas Beklemmendes.»[32] Wie das mittelalterliche «Kinderzeichnen» zielt die Fotografie auf Resurrektion, auf Auferstehung, aber im klaren Bewusstsein ihres eigenen Scheiterns. Fotografien vergehen, ebenso wie die Menschen. Auch davon erzählen die unscharfen Bilder zwischen den «Nicht-Porträts» vom Abschied Chiaras.

1 Vgl. Ernst Bloch: «Über Tod, Unsterblichkeit, Fortdauer». Ein Gespräch mit Siegfried Unseld, 6. 8. 1969, in Königstein / Taunus. In: *Tendenz – Latenz – Utopie.* Frankfurt am Main: Suhrkamp 1978. Seite 308–336; hier: Seite 329.

2 Vgl. Friedrich Nietzsche: «Die Philosophie im tragischen Zeitalter der Griechen». In: *Sämtliche Werke. Kritische Studienausgabe.* Herausgegeben von Giorgio Colli und Mazzino Montinari. Band 1. München / Berlin / New York: dtv / Walter de Gruyter 1980. Seite 799–872; hier: Seite 818. Vgl. auch Martin Heidegger: «Der Spruch des Anaximander». In: *Holzwege.* Frankfurt am Main: Klostermann 1950. Seite 296–343.

3 Vgl. Arthur Schopenhauer: *Die Welt als Wille und Vorstellung.* Zweiter Band. Sämtliche Werke. Herausgegeben von Arthur Hübscher. Band III. Wiesbaden: Brockhaus 1972. Seite 532 f.

4 Vgl. Sigmund Freud: «Zeitgemäßes über Krieg und Tod [1915]». In: *Fragen der Gesellschaft – Ursprünge der Religion.* Studienausgabe. Herausgegeben von Alexander Mitscherlich, Angela Richards und James Strachey. Band IX. Frankfurt am Main: S. Fischer 1974. Seite 32–60; hier: Seite 49.

5 Vgl. Martin Heidegger: *Sein und Zeit.* Tübingen: Max Niemeyer [15]1979. Seite 258.

6 Ebd. Seite 245.

7 Vgl. Johannes von Tepl: *Der Ackermann und der Tod* [XX. Kapitel]. Übersetzt von Felix Genzmer. Stuttgart: Reclam 1984. Seite 36.

8 Vgl. Samuel Beckett: *Warten auf Godot.* Übersetzt von Elmar Tophoven. Frankfurt am Main: Suhrkamp 1960. Seite 111.

9 Vgl. Aristoteles: *Tierkunde VII,* 12. Übersetzt und herausgegeben von Paul Gohlke. Paderborn: Schöningh [2]1957. Seite 322 [588 a 8–10]. Vgl. auch Karl-Heinz Leven (Hg.): *Antike Medizin. Ein Lexikon.* München: C.H. Beck 2005. Spalte 497.

10 Vgl. Edward Shorter: *Der weibliche Körper als Schicksal. Zur Sozialgeschichte der Frau.* Übersetzt von Hainer Kober. München/Zürich: Piper [2]1987. Seite 92 f.

11 Vgl. *Frauenmedizin in der Antike.* Griechisch / Lateinisch / Deutsch. Übersetzt und herausgegeben von Charlotte Schubert und Ulrich Huttner. Düsseldorf / Zürich: Artemis & Winkler 1999. Seite 370–381.

12 Vgl. Novalis: Werke, Tagebücher und Briefe Friedrich von Hardenbergs. Herausgegeben von Hans-Joachim Mähl und Richard Samuel. Band III: Kommentar von Hans Jürgen Balmes. München / Wien: Hanser 1987. Seite 649.

13 Vgl. etwa Philippe Ariès: *Geschichte der Kindheit.* Übersetzt von Caroline Neubaur und Karin Kersten. München / Wien: Hanser [2]1976; vgl. auch *Hört ihr die Kinder weinen. Eine psychogenetische Geschichte der Kindheit.* Herausgegeben von Lloyd de Mause. Übersetzt von Ute Auhagen, Christel Beier, Helga Herborth, Reinhard Kaiser, Renate und Rolf Wiggershaus. Frankfurt am Main: Suhrkamp 1977.

14 Vgl. Jacques Le Goff / Nicolas Truong: *Die Geschichte des Körpers im Mittelalter.* Übersetzt von Renate Warttmann. Stuttgart: Klett-Cotta 2007. Seite 110 f.

15 Vgl. Joseph Groben: *Requiem für ein Kind. Trauer und Trost berühmter Eltern.* Köln: Dittrich 2001. Seite 35.

16 Ebd. Seite 38.

17 Ebd. Seite 37.

18 Vgl. Susi Ulrich-Bochsler / Daniel Gutscher: «Wiedererweckung von Totgeborenen». Ein Schweizer Wallfahrtszentrum im Blick von Archäologie und Anthropologie. In: Jürgen Schlumbohm / Barbara Duden / Jacques Gélis / Patrice Veit (Hg.): *Rituale der Geburt. Eine Kulturgeschichte.* München: C.H. Beck 1998. Seite 244–268; hier: Seite 260.

19 Vgl. Jay Ruby: *Secure the Shadow. Death and Photography in America.* Cambridge (Massachusetts) / London: MIT-Press 1995. Seite 31 f.

20 Vgl. Sylvia Mattl-Wurm: «Wien, wo der Tod auch nicht mehr zu Hause ist». In: *Bilder vom Tod.* Katalog zur 168. Sonderausstellung des Historischen Museums der Stadt Wien (30. Oktober 1992 bis 10. Januar 1993). Wien: Historisches Museum 1992. Seite 51–69; hier: Seite 57. Vgl. auch die Abbildung auf Seite 135.

21 Vgl. Martin Schulz: «Die Sichtbarkeit des Todes in der Fotografie». In: Thomas Macho / Kristin Marek (Hg.): *Die neue Sichtbarkeit des Todes.* München: Wilhelm Fink 2007. Seite 401–425.

22 Vgl. *Geschichte der Fotografie in Österreich.* In zwei Bänden herausgegeben vom Verein zur Erarbeitung der

Geschichte der Fotografie in Österreich. Wien: Museum moderner Kunst 1983. Band I: Seite 23 und 79. Band II: Seite 158.

23 Vgl. Jay Ruby: *Secure the Shadow.* A.a.O. (Anm. 21). Seite 60–85.

24 Vgl. Stanley B. Burns: *Sleeping Beauty. Memorial Photography in America.* Altadena (California): Twelvetrees-Press 1990.

25 Vgl. Philippe Ariès: *Bilder zur Geschichte des Todes.* Übersetzt von Hans-Horst Henschen. München / Wien: Hanser 1984. Seite 264.

26 Vgl. Immanuel Kant: *Anthropologie in pragmatischer Hinsicht.* Herausgegeben von Wolfgang Becker. Stuttgart: Reclam 1983. Seite 87.

27 Vgl. Max Frisch: «Totenrede am 18. Oktober 1982 im Grossmünster in Zürich». In: Peter Noll: *Diktate über Sterben & Tod.* Zürich: pendo 1984. Seite 279–284; hier: Seite 284.

28 Am 2. Juli 2007 hat Charlotte Klonk ihren Vortrag zur Habilitation für das Fach Kunstgeschichte an der Humboldt-Universität Berlin dem Thema «einer kleinen Geschichte des Nicht-Porträts» gewidmet.

29 Vgl. Joseph Groben: *Requiem für ein Kind.* A.a.O. (Anm. 15). Seite 36.

30 Vgl. Stephan Hadraschek: «Trost und Hoffnung». Die Bestattung stillgeborener Kinder – ein Beispiel aus der Berliner Charité. In: *Ewig. Forum für Gedenkkultur.* Heft 3 zum Themenschwerpunkt: Kinder, Tod und Trauer. München: Lothar Fölbach 2006. Seite 16–19.

31 Vgl. Roland Barthes: *Die helle Kammer.* Bemerkungen zur Photographie. Übersetzt von Dietrich Leube. Frankfurt am Main: Suhrkamp 1985. Seite 103.

32 Vgl. Susan Sontag: *Über Fotografie.* Übersetzt von Mark W. Rien und Gertrud Baruch. Frankfurt am Main: Fischer 1980. Seite 72.

Thomas Macho

CHIARA'S FAREWELL OR: ON THE DEATH OF CHILDREN

Anaximander's Proposition

News of the death of a child is devastating. Questions about the lack of sense are practically a reflex reaction: accusations of injustice, feelings that a rule has been broken, that of the chronological arrangement of genealogy. Children should bury their parents, not the other way around. Nowadays, we tend to see statistics pertaining to life expectancy as corresponding with the natural course of life, as though the laws of mortality first apply at a certain age. In this type of perspective, death is always unjust, "a stroke of the ax for most, even when they're old,"[1] as Ernst Bloch stated in a conversation with Siegfried Unseld on the day that Adorno died, a few weeks after Bloch's eighty-fourth birthday. Or is it life itself that is unjust, because it always implicates surviving the countless people who have died? Among the oldest texts of European philosophy is a fragment attributed to the philosopher of nature Anaximander, a reputed student of Thales, meant to have lived in Milet from ca. 610 to 547 a. C. The fragment was most recently handed down from the writings of the neo-Platonic Simplicius (sixth century). Many authors, such as Friedrich Nietzsche and Martin Heidegger, have translated Anaximander's dark verdict: "Where the source of things is, to that place they must also pass away, according to necessity, for they must pay penance and be judged for their injustices, in accordance with the ordinance of time."[2]

It is not easy to interpret this fragment appropriately. Apparently, it claims symmetry of origins and passing, which remotely recalls the Indian Karma teachings, or Christian theology of the deadly sins; it speaks of an ordinance of time, of injustice and punishment. Death is derived from birth, but not in the sense of Schopenhauer, who poses the question of why the time before birth frightens us less than the time of non-existence after death.[3] An injustice seems to be at the core, which must be atoned for in death—a guilt that has to be settled. But who are the creditors? Ancestors and forefathers? A great mother? A God who created the world and humanity? Nature, which—as Freud critically surmised—"every one of us" believes to owe a death.[4] Or is it the things themselves that must atone for their original break with *apeiron*, the boundlessness? According to which rules? Even less clear than the question of to whom this guilt is addressed is the question of the criteria for gratification: Anaximander's recourse to the ordinance of time. Which time and which ordinance? Records from the calendar or the generations? Cycles of days and nights, seasons, the stars and their conjunctions? Lists of names, births and deaths? The talk of time's ordinance suggests that mortal beings—whether stars or people—are allocated a span of time that cannot be increased. And when this span of time isn't even exhausted?

The end can occur prematurely. The sun can darken in the morning; children can die young. Indeed, every person is mortal, but what unites them, divides them at the same time. For death is certain, but its occurrence undefined; only *that* we have to die is definite, not *how*, *where*, or *when*. "Along with the certainty of death goes the *indefiniteness* of its 'when,'" emphasized Heidegger in § 52 of *Being and Time*;[5] precisely the difference between certainty and indefiniteness presses death, as existence's "most inherent possibility," before our inner eye. The "being-toward-death" is not guaranteed a specific age; the only possible answer to the horror of premature death is claimed by the unity of death and birth. Heidegger quotes from the argument between the Bohemian Ploughman and Death: "Death is a way to be, which

Dasein takes over as soon as it is. 'As soon as a man comes to life, he is old enough to die.'"[6] Naturally, Heidegger conceals here that the dialogue he is quoting is spoken by Death: "…every human owes the debt of death and has inherited death. If you weep for your wife's youth, you are wrong to do so; as soon as a human has life, so soon is he old enough to die."[7] With these words, death appoints itself as donor of life, midwife and grave-digger in one. "Astride of a grave and a difficult birth," comments Vladimir in Samuel Beckett's *Waiting for Godot*: "Down in the hole, lingeringly, the grave-digger puts on the forceps."[8]

Mors immatura

Vladimir's comments are directed at a Western audience in the second half of the twentieth century, in other epochs and cultures they would have probably drawn little attention. *Mors immatura*, premature death, is among one of the most widespread plagues: in Germany, as late as 1870, 250 of every 1,000 children died before reaching their fifth birthday. By 1910 this figure sank to 160, in 1927 it was under 100 for the first time, and by 1970 at approximately 25; in 2006, infant mortality in Germany affected 3.8 of 1,000 children. Accurate, statistically analyzable data are largely missing for past eras. It is estimated, however, that in the Middle Ages and the early years of modernity, only half of an age group survived past the age of twenty-one. Also in classical antiquity, infant mortality was so high that Aristotle could claim, for example, that it is customary and sensible to first give the newborn child a name after the course of a week, "from a belief that it has now a better chance of survival."[9] The main causes of children's deaths were too little or improper nutrition, infections, and diseases (such as tuberculosis) or serious complications at birth: transverse, breech, or occiput positions of the fetus. Indeed, such cases occurred only for approximately 4 percent of all births, but they always meant a considerable threat to the life of the mother and the child,[10] which could only be dealt with by unusual methods—such as the infamous embryotomy, the dismemberment of the fetus in the womb.[11]

The statistics must be made concrete. Long before painting his gruesome Saturn (1820–1823), Spanish painter Francisco de Goya fathered twenty-four children with Josefa Bayeu. One single son, Xavier, survived. In one edition of the works of Count Friedrich von Hardenberg, better known by his penname Novalis, there is a family tree, a simple compilation of the names and dates which constituted a family two-hundred years ago;[12] from this, it is evident that Novalis, himself, died on 25 March 1801 when he was twenty-nine years old. Of his ten siblings, only two brothers lived to be older than thirty—Carl and Georg Anton, who at thirty-seven and forty-four also did not exactly reach a biblical age. In 1818—the year his mother died—not only had his father already died four years earlier, but also, only one son of eleven children was still alive. And just a remark on the side: the poet's fiancé, Sophie von Kühn, died two days after her fifteenth birthday. The poet Friedrich Rückert lost his two youngest children, Luise und Ernst, within just a few weeks—on 31 December 1833 and on 16 January 1834—to scarlet fever; he then wrote the *Kindertotenlieder*, which Gustav Mahler set to music in 1901 and 1904. Giuseppe Verdi's entire family—daughter and son, at the age of sixteen months, and then his wife—died within two years, between 1838 and 1840. And finally, the Czech composer Antonin Dvořák began work on his great oratorio *Stabat Mater* in mourning for his daughter Josefa (she died on 19 December 1875, two days after birth), yet before completion of this work on 13 November 1877, both his eleven-month old daughter Ruzena and three-year old son Otakar (in August 1877) had died.

It is difficult to empathize with someone who suffered and survived such a sequence of farewells. Therefore, it comes as no surprise that some historians support the opinion that the value of a child's life was not very high in older cultures;[13] it was only the earliest modern era that gradually learned to mourn for deceased children. Such suppositions are difficult to disprove;[14] however, they can be made somewhat relative on the basis of individual examples. For example, after the death of his two-year-old daughter Timoxena, Plutarch wrote a letter of consolation to his wife, in which he emphasized that he was born neither of "a stock nor a stone," but rather, that he knew her pain: "This daughter was born after four sons, when you were longing to bear a daughter; which made me call her by your own name. Therefore I know she was particularly dear to you. And grief must have a peculiar pungency in a mind tenderly affectionate to children, when you call to mind how naturally witty and innocent she was, void of anger, and not querulous."[15] Plutarch believed in the immortality of the soul. In the letter to his wife, he underscored that the laws did not allow them "to lament for those whose souls pass immediately into a better and more divine state,"[16] while at the same time assuring her: "But as long as she is gone to a place where she feels no pain, what need is there of our grief?"[17] Roughly 1,500 years later, Michel de Montaigne sent a translation of this letter of condolence to his own wife, when he received the news of his oldest daughter's death.

Post-mortem pictures of children

According to Christian tradition, the baptism of a child, his or her integration into the church, is considered more important than health or a long life. Heavenly salvation was at stake, and the future abode of the immortal soul. Should the child die shortly after birth—which happened often enough—it was then possible to make one's way to the next church and ask a miraculous image of Maria or a saint to "mark" the child; it was necessary to recognize every brief moment that the baby was called back to life based on visible signs (such as reddened cheeks, breathing noises, or little convulsions), to then quickly perform a christening. The former Marienkapelle in Oberbüren in the Canton of Bern was a well-known center in Switzerland where deceased children could be "brought to life" again in this way. Bishop Otto von Sonnenberg († 1491) described the practice in the following words: The "women warm the dead children between glowing coals and candles and lights placed around them in a circle. A very light feather is placed over the mouths of the warmed-up dead children or premature births and when the feather moves away from the lips, by chance, due to the air or the warmth of the coals, the women claim that the children and premature births have breathed and lived, and immediately have them christened with the ringing of bells and paeans of praise. They then give the body of the child who supposedly came alive and to then immediately die again, a Christian burial."[18] The Marienkapelle was torn down during the Reformation and first examined archeologically just a few years ago. In this, the "Chilchmatt" was uncovered, a burial grounds of more than 3,500 square meters, which had already been used since the Bronze Age. In several places, the archeologists discovered grave areas for more than 250 children who died shortly after birth and were apparently christened at the moment of their brief "re-awakening," as can be assumed by the body positions of the tiny skeletons with their crossed arms and placement in the grave towards Jerusalem.

The "post-mortem portraying of children" shapes a religious practice that was gradually forgotten; only because of such forgetting could accusations be made that medieval parents did not mourn for their dead children. In the emerging era of secularization and criticism of religion, spiritual consolation, which often could no longer be bestowed convincingly, was replaced by artistic forms of expression of grief. The dead children were now actually drawn or painted: Charles Willson Peale, for example, painted his wife and deceased daughter Margaret as *Rachel Weeping* (1772–1776);[19] Viennese painter Friedrich von Amerling portrayed his wife Antonie on her deathbed in 1843, and also seven years later, their son Fritz.[20] After the invention of photography, studios developed in major cities of North America and Europe, which—commonly in cooperation with the cemetery administration and the respective burial institutions—produced the final images of the dead: as a keepsake and memento, and later also as an element on the gravestone.[21] In 1850, Félix Nadar, pioneer of the daguerreotype, offered to take photos of a dead loved-one in his Parisian studio. In Munich, Adolph Scheuerer advertised in 1858 for new commissions for his corpse portraits, with the promise of "greatest possible similarity," and a "friendly expression"; on the Südfriedhof in Munich, by 1857 already more than three hundred of the dead had been photographed in an open casket. In Vienna's Nussdorf, photographer Albin Mutterer, who was the first to build a glass-covered studio, achieved success as a specialist in the new genre of photographing the dead.[22]

In his study on *Death and Photography in America*, Jay Ruby differentiated between several types of depiction of the dead in the nineteenth century: the "Alive, yet dead" pictures, which depicted the deceased in an upright position, often with touched-up eyes; the "Last Sleep" pictures that show the dead as though they were sleeping—for example, on a bed couch or in a cradle—and finally, the photographs of the dead in an open casket.[23] In numerous pictures, one sees the relatives of the dead, in some cases all of the mourners, which in any case refutes the cynical aperçu, whereby the older photographs with their long exposure times favored portraits of the dead because corpses do not blur any picture. Most of the photos of the dead collected by Jay Ruby (or Stanley B. Burns[24]), present, by the way, deceased children; Philippe Ariès accurately points out: "Every family album contained photos of dead children ..." He explains that the death of a child is the first unbearable death. Children's grave stones did not exist before the sixteenth century or were unusual. In the seventeenth century, they remained seldom and gauche. In the nineteenth century, on the contrary, the children literally conquered the cemeteries. "Parents evidently desired to represent their dead children in all kinds of attitudes in order to express their intense grief and their passionate desire to make their children survive in memory and in art, to exalt the children's innocence, charm, and beauty."[25]

Chiara's Farewell

There is no trace of such "enthusiastic excess" in the photos that Elisabeth Zahnd Legnazzi took of her daughter Chiara during the child's slow death. The sequence of images witnesses the child's departure, a gradual retreat from the world: visible is the gaze that no longer finds a vis-à-vis. In his *Anthropology from a Pragmatic Point of View* (1798), Immanuel Kant defined death as the end point in a number of losses of the sense faculties, whereby drunkenness is associated with sleep, and unconsciousness with apparent death (asphyxia), as "foretaste" of death. But he also emphasized the insurmountable state that separates the most extreme unconsciousness from the actual entry of death. "No human being can experience his own *death* (for to constitute an experience requires life), he can only observe it in others."[26] I can see that I am no longer seen; in that is the deepest injury that can be inflicted on the survivors. In his funeral oration for Peter Noll, Max Frisch remarked on 18 October 1982: "We are gathered together to mourn. Ignorant of what death is, the common expression of our genuine grief is to publicly praise a deceased man and publicly declare that one will miss him. Never have I seen a face in a casket that has shown me that those who have just died miss us. The opposite is clearly obvious ... The dead person leaves us alone with the memories of our times together ..."[27]

In the transition from sleeping to waking, Chiara does not seem to see that she is seen and photographed. On the contrary, she seems to see what the photographer is unable to see. In this way, the child's face withdraws from any temptation to pose. It advances to a "non-portrait" (to refer to an expression by Charlotte Klonk[28]). A "non-portrait" breaks the contract of representation: the promise of a visualized presence that is experienced as a *shared* time between the observer and the observed. Yet a face that seems not to see that it is seen, what does it show? It does not demonstrate its own absence, but rather, the absence of the other. Thus, it becomes even more urgent to accompany her: in a few cases by her father or mother, sometimes by flowers or a stuffed animal. In the end, the flowers and the gallery of stuffed animals—no less touching than human mourners—hold watch over the dead girl. Why are we unsettled by the presence of precisely these things? Why did Plutarch implore his dead daughter, "compassionate to miracle," by recalling how the child "...would pray her nurse to give suck, not only to other children, but to her very playthings, as it were courteously inviting them to her table, and making the best cheer for them she could."[29] Things are media of transformation, bridges between people and the material world; commonly it is playthings that accompany children into the grave as the last gifts, or decorate their graves.[30]

Between the "non-portrait" of the young girl Chiara (literally: the gleaming, the bright one—further emphasized by her middle name: *Lucia*, the luminous, the light) appear several blurry photos whose objects—colored surfaces, points of light, interior and exterior spaces—cannot be clearly recognized. The large-format images, which do not depict anything, refer to the child's failing eyesight; but they can also be related to that *Journey into Light* announced in the book's subtitle. This subtitle refers, on the one hand, to those commonly quoted near-death reports that seem to depict a birth experience of sorts: a journey through a tunnel at the end of which one perceives a radiant light. On the other hand, however, it refers to the essence of photography itself. Since its invention, the art of recording light images has been associated with death. Roland Barthes wrote, in this sense, of the horror of death, that there is "nothing to say about the death of one whom I love most, nothing to say about her photograph, which I contemplate without ever being able to get to the heart of it, to transform it."[31] For death is as contingent as every moment that photography lends permanent shape. "Photography is the inventory of mortality," remarked Susan Sontag. "Photographs state the innocence, the vulnerability of lives headed toward their own destruction, and this link between photography and death haunts all photographs of people."[32] Like the medieval "drawings of children," photography aims at resurrection, at rebirth, but remains clearly aware of its own failure. Photographs die, just like people do. Telling of this, too, are the blurry pictures between the "non-portraits" of Chiara's farewell.

1 See Ernst Bloch, "Über Tod, Unsterblichkeit, Fortdauer. Ein Gespräch mit Siegfried Unseld, 6. 8. 1969, in Königstein / Taunus," in *Tendenz – Latenz – Utopie,* Frankfurt am Main: Suhrkamp, 1978, pp. 308–336; here, p. 329.

2 See Friedrich Nietzsche, *Philosophy in the Tragic Age of the Greeks*, transl. Marianne Cowan, Washington D.C.: Regnery Publishing, 1996, p. 45. See also Martin Heidegger, "Anaximander's Saying," in *Off the Beaten Track*, Cambridge: University of Cambridge Press, 2002, p. 242.

3 See Arthur Schopenhauer, *The World as Will and Idea*, transl. R. B. Haldane, J. Kemp, New York: AMS Press, 1977, p. 254.

4 See Sigmund Freud, "Thoughts for the Times on War and Death," in *The Standard Edition of the Complete Psychological Works of Sigmund Freud,* Vol. IV., London: Hogarth Press, 1953.

5 See Martin Heidegger, *Being and Time,* transl. John Macquarrie and Edward Robinson, New York: Harper and Row, 1962, p. 302.

6 Ibid., p. 289.

7 See Johannes von Tepl, *Der Ackermann und der Tod.* For a modern English translation see chapter 20, http://www.michaelhaldane.com/Husbandmanand-Death. Also translated by Michael West as *Death and the Ploughman*, London: A&C Black, 2003.

8 See Samuel Beckett, *Waiting for Godot,* New York: Grove Press, 1994 (first published 1954), p. 104.

9 See Aristotle, *The History of Animals, VII, 12,* transl. D'Arcy Wentworth Thompson, University of Adelaide, South Australia: http://ebooks.adelaide.edu.au/a/aristotle/history/, 2007. See also Karl-Heinz Leven (ed.), *Antike Medizin. Ein Lexikon*, Munich: C.H. Beck, 2005, column 497.

10 See Edward Shorter, *Women's Bodies: A Social History of Women's Encounter with Health, Ill-health, and Medicine*, Edison, NJ: Transaction Publishers, 1991, p. 74.

11 See *Frauenmedizin in der Antike.* Griechisch / Lateinisch / Deutsch, ed. and transl. by Charlotte Schubert and Ulrich Huttner, Düsseldorf / Zürich: Artemis & Winkler, 1999, pp. 370–381.

12 See Novalis: *Werke, Tagebücher und Briefe Friedrich von Hardenbergs,* eds. Hans-Joachim Mähl and Richard Samuel, Vol. III: Commentary by Hans Jürgen Balmes, Munich / Vienna: Hanser, 1987, p. 649.

13 See, for example, Philippe Ariès, *Centuries of Childhood: A Social History of Family Life*, transl. Robert Baldick, New York: Random House, 1962; see also ed. Lloyd DeMause, *The History of Childhood*, New York: Harper, 1974.

14 See Jacques Le Goff / Nicolas Truong, *Une histoire du corps au Moyen Âge*, Paris: L. Levi, 2003.

15 See *Plutarch's Morals, Translated from the Greek by Several Hands. Corrected and Revised by William W. Goodwin, with an Introduction by Ralph Waldo Emerson,* 5 Volumes, Boston: Little, Brown, and Co., 1878, Vol. 5: "Plutarch's Consolatory Letter to His Wife".

16 Ibid.

17 Ibid.

18 See Susi Ulrich-Bochsler and Daniel Gutscher, "Wiedererweckung von Totgeborenen. Ein Schweizer Wallfahrtszentrum im Blick von Archäologie und Anthropologie," in eds. Jürgen Schlumbohm, Barbara Duden, Jacques Gélis, and Patrice Veit, *Rituale der Geburt. Eine Kulturgeschichte*, Munich: C.H. Beck, 1998, pp. 244–268; here, p. 260.

19 See Jay Ruby, *Secure the Shadow. Death and Photography in America*, Cambridge (Mass) / London: MIT-Press, 1995, p. 31 f.

20 See Sylvia Mattl-Wurm, "Wien, wo der Tod auch nicht mehr zu Hause ist," in *Bilder vom Tod.* Catalogue for the 168th special exhibition of the Historical Museum of the City of Vienna (30 October 1992 to 10 January 1993), Vienna: Historical Museum, 1992, pp. 51–69; here, p. 57, see also the illustration on page 135.

21 See Martin Schulz, "Die Sichtbarkeit des Todes in der Fotografie," in eds. Thomas Macho and Kristin Marek, *Die neue Sichtbarkeit des Todes,* Munich: Wilhelm Fink, 2007, pp. 401–425.

22 See *Geschichte der Fotografie in Österreich,* published in two volumes by the Verein zur Erarbeitung der Geschichte der Fotografie in Österreich, Vienna: Museum of Modern Art (MUMOK), 1983, Vol. I, pp. 23 and 79, Vol. II, p. 158.

23 See note 19, Jay Ruby, *Secure the Shadow* (on the cited page, note 21), pp. 60–85.

24 See Stanley B. Burns, *Sleeping Beauty. Memorial Photography in America*, Altadena (California): Twelvetrees-Press, 1990.

25 See Philippe Ariès, *Images of Man and Death,* transl. Janet Lloyd, Cambridge, MA: Harvard University Press, 1985. p. 252

26 See Immanuel Kant, *Anthropology from a Pragmatic Point of View,* Cambridge: Cambridge University Press, 2006, p. 59.

27 See Max Frisch, "Totenrede am 18. Oktober 1982 im Grossmünster in Zürich," in Peter Noll, *Diktate über Sterben & Tod,* Zürich: pendo, 1984, pp. 279–284; here p. 284.

28 On 2 July 2007, Charlotte Klonk devoted her lecture for habilitation in Art History at Humboldt University Berlin to the theme "einer kleinen Geschichte des Nicht-Porträts" (A brief history of the non-portrait).

29 See "Plutarch's Consolatory Letter to his Wife," see note 15.

30 See Stephan Hadraschek, "Trost und Hoffnung. Die Bestattung stillgeborener Kinder – ein Beispiel aus der Berliner Charité," in *Ewig. Forum für Gedenkkultur,* no. 3 with a focus on: Kinder, Tod und Trauer, Munich: Lothar Fölbach, 2006, pp. 16–19.

31 See Roland Barthes, *Camera Lucida: Reflections on Photography*, transl: Richard Howard, New York: Hill and Wang, 1981, p. 93.

32 See Susan Sontag, *On Photography*, New York: Picador, 1973, p. 70.

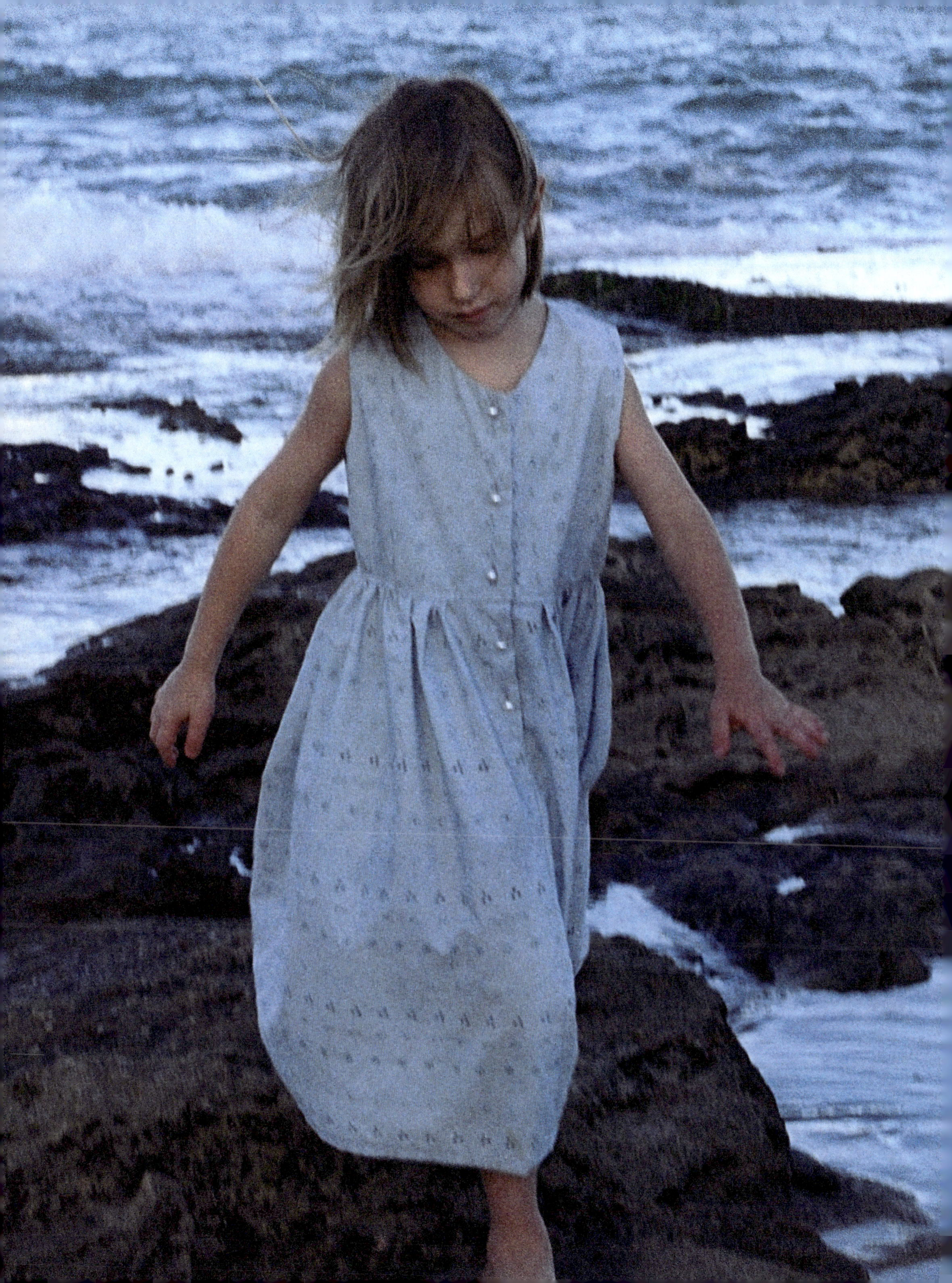

Ich danke meinem Mann Remo Legnazzi, seinen Schwestern Isabelle und Manuela, meiner lieben Mutter, Dr. Andreas Giger, Dr. Bernhard Wingeier, dem Team der Familienstation der Ita Wegman Klinik, Lis Winiger, Katrin Wirz, Katharina Gusset und Max Roth, Jangchub Iseli-Songma, Laurence und Orm Bonsma-Reist für ihre Anteilnahme und Hilfe sowie allen Verwandten, Freunden, Nachbarn und Nachbarskindern, die uns unterstützt haben. Besonderen Dank geht an Peter Erismann, ohne den das Buch so nicht zustande gekommen wäre.

I thank my husband Remo Legnazzi, his sisters Isabelle and Manuela, my dear mother, Dr. Andreas Giger, Dr. Bernhard Wingeier, the team of the family station at the Ita Wegman Clinic, Lis Winiger, Katrin Wirz, Katharina Gusset and Max Roth, Jangchub Iseli-Songma, and Laurence and Orm Bonsma-Reist for their compassion and help as well as all relatives, friends, neighbors and their children who supported us. Special thanks go to Peter Erismann, without whom the book would not have been possible.

Fondation Janyce   Fondation Johanna Dürmüller-Bol
Jubiläumsstiftung der Zürich Versicherungsgruppe
Kanton Bern   Palliative Care – Netzwerk Kanton Bern
Reformierte Kirchen Bern – Jura – Solothurn   Reformierte Landeskirche des Kantons Zürich   S. Eustachius Stiftung
Schweizerische Gesellschaft für Palliative Medizin (SGPMP)
Stadt Bern   Stiftung Pro Pallium

Der Anblick von Schwerkranken erinnert uns immer auch an die eigene Sterblichkeit. Doch wie der Volksmund sagt: Das einzig Sichere im Leben ist der Tod. Früher oder später sterben wir alle. Der Tod und die damit verbundene Angst vor den bevorstehenden Leiden haben allerdings in unserer modernen Leistungsgesellschaft keinen Platz und werden, so gut es geht, verdrängt. Furcht ist jedoch ein schlechter Wegbegleiter in den Tod. Befasst man sich mit dieser Angst und setzt sich frühzeitig mit dem Tod auseinander, verliert er seinen Schrecken. Genauso wichtig wie die Vorbereitung auf den eigenen Tod ist es, anderen beizustehen: So wie Eltern mit ihrer Liebe und Fürsorge dem hilflosen Neugeborenen helfen, in der unbekannten neuen Welt Fuss zu fassen, können wir auch mit Liebe und Mitgefühl den hilflosen Sterbenden begleiten und versuchen, ihm ein friedliches und würdevolles Sterben zu ermöglichen.

The sight of the terminally ill always reminds us of our own mortality. Yet, as the saying goes: the only thing certain about life is death. Sooner or later, we all die. Yet death and the fear of imminent suffering that goes along with it have no place in our modern achievement-based society, and are suppressed as much as possible. Dread, however, is not the best companion on the way to death. If one addresses this fear and confronts death early on, the horror vanishes. Just as important as preparing for one's own death, is assisting others: In the same way that parents, with their love and care, help the defenseless newborn gain footing in the unknown new world, we can also accompany those who are defenselessly passing away by attempting to permit them a peaceful and dignified death.

Elisabeth Zahnd Legnazzi

Elisabeth Zahnd Legnazzi

geboren 1957 in Bern, machte eine Ausbildung zur Fotografin (1974–1977) und an der Schule für Gestaltung Bern (heute Hochschule der Künste) eine Weiterbildung im Bereich Videofilm (1994–1996). Sie ist seit 1983 freischaffende Künstlerin und hat ihre Fotografien, Videoarbeiten und Installationen an Einzel- und Gruppenausstellungen gezeigt, u. a. in der Kunsthalle Bern (1984), im Kunstmuseum Bern (1987, 2005), im Kulturzentrum Kammgarn Schaffhausen (1991), in der Kunsthalle Winterthur (1993), im Kunsthaus Langenthal (1994), in Joao Pessoa, Brasilien (1998), der Galerie Kunstkeller Bern (1999) und im Zentrum für Kulturproduktion PROGR, Bern (2008). Elisabeth Zahnd realisierte auch Kunst am Bau-Projekte und erhielt mehrere Stipendien und Auszeichnungen, unter anderem das Atelierstipendium Paris (1987), Projektbeiträge von Stadt und Kanton Bern und einen Werkbeitrag der Kantonalen Kommission für Foto und Film (2002). Sie lebt mit ihrem Mann und ihrem Sohn in Bern und in Salvador da Bahia, Brasilien.

Thomas Macho

geboren 1952 in Wien, ist Kulturwissenschaftler, Philosoph und Professor für Kulturgeschichte an der Humboldt-Universität in Berlin. Er studierte Philosophie, Musikwissenschaft und Pädagogik und promovierte 1976 mit einer Dissertation zur Philosophie der Musik. 1983 folgte die Habilitation im Fach Philosophie mit der Schrift *Von den Metaphern des Todes. Eine Phänomenologie der Grenzerfahrung*. Thomas Macho forscht u. a. zur Geschichte der Zeitrechnung, über Tod und Totenkulte. Er war u. a. Mitbegründer des Hermann von Helmholtz-Zentrums für Kulturtechnik an der Humboldt-Universität Berlin (1999), Preisträger der Aby-Warburg-Stiftung (2001), Prodekan (2003–2005) und Dekan (2006–2008) der Philosophischen Fakultät III der Humboldt-Universität. Seine jüngsten Publikationen sind *Tiefenrausch – Ein Lesebuch zur Unterwelt* (Folio Verlag, Wien 2008), *Zwei Grad. Das Wetter, der Mensch und sein Klima* (Wallstein Verlag, Göttingen 2008) und, gemeinsam mit Kristin Marek, *Die neue Sichtbarkeit des Todes* (Wilhelm Fink Verlag, München 2007). Thomas Macho schreibt regelmässig auch für die *Neue Zürcher Zeitung* und *Die Zeit*. Er lebt in Berlin.

Nadine Olonetzky

geboren 1962 in Zürich, schreibt als freie Autorin für die *NZZ am Sonntag*, Zeitschriften und Bücher zu Themen aus Fotografie, Kunst und Kulturgeschichte (www.kontrast.ch) und ist Lektorin im Verlag Scheidegger & Spiess, Zürich.

Elisabeth Zahnd Legnazzi

born in Bern in 1957, was trained as a photographer (1974–1977) and continued her education at the Schule für Gestaltung Bern (today, Bern University of the Arts) in the area of video (1994–1996). She has been a freelance artist since 1983 and has shown her photographs, videos, and installations in solo and group exhibitions, at the Kunsthalle Bern (1984), Museum of Fine Arts Bern (1987, 2005), Culture Center Kammgarn Schaffhausen (1991), Kunsthalle Winterthur (1993), Kunsthaus Langenthal (1994), Joao Pessoa, Brazil (1998), Galerie Kunstkeller Bern (1999), and at the Zentrum für Kulturproduktion PROGR, Bern (2008). Elisabeth Zahnd has also realized art and architecture projects and has been awarded several grants and honors, including a studio grant Paris (1987). She has contributed to projects for the City of Bern and Canton of Bern and contributed a work to the Canton Commission for Photo and Film (2002). She lives with her husband and son in Bern and in Salvador da Bahia, Brazil.

Thomas Macho

born in Vienna in 1952, is a cultural studies scholar, philosopher, and professor of cultural history at the Humboldt University in Berlin. He studied philosophy, musicology, and education science and received his doctorate in 1976 with a dissertation on the philosophy of music. In 1983 he wrote his habilitation in philosophy, *Von den Metaphern des Todes. Eine Phänomenologie der Grenzerfahrung*. Thomas Macho's research includes the history of the computation of time, death, and death cults. He was, among other things, co-founder of the Hermann von Helmholtz-Zentrum für Kulturtechnik at Humboldt University Berlin (1999), winner of the Aby-Warburg-Stiftung (2001), vice dean (2003–2005) and dean (2006–2008) of the philosophy department III at Humboldt University. His most recent publications are *Tiefenrausch – Ein Lesebuch zur Unterwelt* (Folio Verlag, Vienna 2008), *Zwei Grad. Das Wetter, der Mensch und sein Klima* (Wallstein Verlag, Göttingen 2008) and, together with Kristin Marek, *Die neue Sichtbarkeit des Todes* (Wilhelm Fink Verlag, Munich 2007). Thomas Macho writes regularly for the *Neue Zürcher Zeitung* and *Die Zeit*. He lives in Berlin.

Nadine Olonetzky

born in Zurich 1962, is a freelance author contributing to *NZZ am Sonntag*, magazines, and books on themes related to photography, art, and cultural history (www.kontrast.ch) and is an editor at Verlag Scheidegger & Spiess, Zurich.

Konzept / Concept:
Elisabeth Zahnd Legnazzi

Texte / Texts:
Thomas Macho, Nadine Olonetzky

Lektorat deutsch / Copyediting German:
Thomas Kramer, Nadine Olonetzky

Übersetzung / Translation:
Lisa Rosenblatt, Wien / Vienna

Korrektorat deutsch und englisch / Proofreading German and English: Claudia Mazanek, Wien / Vienna

Gestaltung / Design:
Elisabeth Zahnd Legnazzi mit / with
Franziska Schott & Marco Schibig, Bern

Lithografien, Druck und Bindung / Lithographs, printing, and binding: DZA Druckerei zu Altenburg GmbH, D-Altenburg

ISBN 978-3-85881-238-4

Verlag Scheidegger & Spiess AG, Zürich
Niederdorfstrasse 54
CH-8001 Zürich

www.scheidegger-spiess.ch